MORE INSTANT TEACHING TOOLS

FOR

HEALTH CARE EDUCATORS

Michele L. Deck, MEd, BSN, RN, ACCE-R

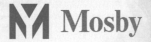 Mosby

St. Louis Baltimore Boston Carlsbad Chicago Naples New York Philadelphia Portland
London Madrid Mexico City Singapore Sydney Tokyo Toronto Wiesbaden

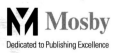

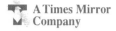

Vice President and Publisher Nancy L. Coon
Editor: Barry Bowlus
Developmental Editor: Barbara Watts
Project Manager: Gayle Morris
Editing, Production and Design: Graphic World Publishing Services
Manufacturing Manager: Betty Mueller

Printed in the United States of America

Composition by Graphic World, Inc.

Printing/binding by R. R. Donnelley and Sons Company

Mosby–Year Book, Inc.

11830 Westline Industrial Drive

St. Louis, Missouri 63146

International Standard Book Number 0-323-00085-1

97 98 99 00 / 9 8 7 6 5 4 3 2 1

Michele Deck
MEd, BSN, RN, ACCE-R

Michele is known for her innovative teaching methods in the field of health care education. In February 1989 the Journal of Pediatric Nursing published her article "The Games We Play." In May 1990 Creative Training Techniques published her manual *Getting Adults Motivated, Enthusiastic and Satisfied,* based on her experience using television game shows as a method of instruction for technical information. She has been cited with her co-author Jeanne R. Silva in eight separate issues of *Creative Training Techniques Newsletter,* an internationally circulated newsletter by Lakewood Publications. Her four latest books are *Instant Teaching Tools For Healthcare Educators; Presenter's Survival Kit: It's A Jungle Out There!; Getting Adults Motivated, Enthusiastic and Satisfied Volume Two;* and *The Presenter's E-Z Graphics Kit: A Guide For The Artistically Challenged.* Michele is also owner of G.A.M.E.S. (Gimics And Mania Educate Staff), a Nursing Education Consulting firm in Metairie, Louisiana. Her latest venture is a creative product company called Tool Thyme for Trainers, which features items to make repetitive sessions fun for all.

In 1992 Michele presented at the American Society for Training and Development's (ASTD) national conference. She conducted a preconference session at the 1991 national American Society for Healthcare Education and Training (ASHET) and was one of the highest-rated speakers. Michele has presented throughout the United States, Canada, and Europe. She has presented at Mosby's staff development conference annually since 1992. Allegheny University has invited Michele to present several years in a row at both the Nursing Staff Development Conference and Faculty Development Conferences. Michele has been on the national faculty of many conferences. In 1994, she presented a preconference for the national meeting of the American Association of Critical Care Nurses and congress sessions at the National Association of Operating Room Nurses and the National Association of Orthopaedic Nurses. The American Association of Office Nurses invited her in 1994 and 1995. In 1995, 1996, and 1997 she presented at the national conferences of the Emergency Nurses Association. The American Association of Operating Room Nurses had her back in 1997. She consistently receives high evaluations for her fun, informative, and idea-filled sessions.

Contributors

Jeri L. Ashley, MSN, RN, AOCN
Memphis, TN

Julia W. Aucoin, MN, RN,C
Faculty
North Carolina Central
University Department of
Nursing
Durham, NC

Sherry L. Blanchard, RN
Nurse Aide Instructor
Wever, IA

Pamela Brown Stewart, MN, RN, CCRN
Impact Education
Ellicott, MD

Mary Arnone Cahoon, BS, RN
Staff Development and Training
Coordinator Health Services
Community Health and
Counseling Services
Bangor, ME

Linda Chitwood, MS, RN
Louise Alice School of Nursing
Suffolk, VA

Sandra H. Clark, MSN, RN
Savannah, GA

Teresa Colgan, BSN, RN
Burlington Medical Center
Burlington, IA

Erin E. Davis, MS, MEd, RRT
Director of Clinical Education
Program in Respiratory Care
Ochsner School of Allied
Health Sciences
New Orleans, LA

Terry Delpier, MN, RN, CPNP
Assistant Professor of
Nursing, Pediatrics
Northern Michigan University
Marquette, MI

Susan Duly, BSN, CNOR, RN
Clinical Education Specialist
Surgical Care Center
Parkview Memorial Hospital
Fort Wayne, IN

Ann Eubanks, RN, CCRN
Critical Care Clinician
Springhill Memorial Hospital
Mobile, AL

Janet Fitts, BSN, RN, CEN,TNS, EMT-P
Trauma Nurse Coordinator
St John's Mercy Hospital
Washington, MO
Paramedic Instructor
East Central College
Union, MO

Elaine Frank, MHS
Program Director
Injury Prevention Center
Dartmouth-Hitchcock
Medical Center
Hanover, NH

Penny Gorman, BSN, RN
Clinical Education Specialist
Surgical Care Center
Parkview Memorial Hospital
Fort Wayne, IN

Kathy Harding, MSN, RN
Instructor of Nursing
West Texas A&M University
Canyon, TX

continued

Contributors *continued*

Nancy Hennen, BSN, RNC
Clinical Educator
Ochsner Foundation Hospital
New Orleans, LA

Elaine Hinojosa, MN, RNC
Clinical Educator
Ochsner Foundation Hospital
New Orleans, LA

Mary Ann Jones, MA, RN
Founder
American Association
of Office Nurses
Montvale, NJ

Fran Kelly
Springhill Memorial Hospital
Mobile, AL

Mary LaBiche, MEd, RRT
Program Director
Program in Respiratory Care
Ochsner School of Allied Health
Sciences
New Orleans, LA

Lynn Lippitt
NH Housing Authority
Bedford, NH

Jana Magarelli, MA, RN
Clinical Instructor, Critical Care
Hackensack University
Medical Center
Hackensack, NJ

Nancy Moulaison, BSN, RN
Nursing Instructor/Education
Consultant
Sanford Brown College
St Louis, MO

Bernadette Price, RN, MSN
Associate Professor of Nursing
Purdue University, Calumet
Hammond, IN

Chris Reid, RN, MSN
Associate Professor of Nursing
Purdue University, Calumet
Hammond, IN

**Jeanne R. Silva, BSN,
RN, CCRN**
Consultant
Gimics And Mania
Educate Staff
Metairie, LA

**Mary Beth Swaboda, MSN,
RN, CCRN**
Critical Care Educator
Methodist Hospital
San Antonio, TX

Hal Vizino
Education Coordinator
Parkview Memorial Hospital
Fort Wayne, IN

Tom Wilson
Springhill Memorial Hospital
Mobile, AL

**Sandra L. Woodbury, MS,
RN, CCRN**
Clinical Instructor
Morton College
Hinsdale, IL

Reviewers

Donna Streater Bates, RNC, MSN
Nursing Programs Manager
Hospital Education
Duke University Medical Center
Durham, NC

Amelia Griffin, RN, MSN
Director of Nursing Education
Wake AHEC
Raleigh, NC

Carolyn Russett, RNC, BSN, OCN
Coordinator, Staff Development
Cape Cod Hospital
Hyannis, MA

Preface

Welcome aboard! You are invited to enjoy the journey to teaching healthcare content in a variety of innovative ways. To those of you who began this journey with *Instant Teaching Tools for Health Care Educators,* let me welcome you as you reboard for the continuation of a lovely trip. For those new travelers, let me invite you to enjoy the journey through this book of discovery.

This book is gathered from health care educators who know there are many ways to teach content. Maybe it is your quest for a new road yourself that has led you here to this book. Maybe you just happened to board by accident. Whatever your reason for picking up this book, it provides something that is difficult to find: instant ways to teach health care content creatively. A group of determined and skilled health care educators found a new and innovative approach that worked and were willing to share it here with you and me.

The book is written so that you can either sample it or enjoy a long and satisfying trip. It is not necessary to read the entire book to obtain an idea that you can use in your next educational session. Think of your audience, and select one that you suspect they will like because you like it yourself!

Health care educators are the key to learning. Our enjoyment of content delivery is contagious. If we feel like it is a drudge or chore to be endured, our audience will get that message loudly and clearly. Even if we never say negative words, our body language and our attitude are the biggest messages learners receive. Over eighty percent of our message is taken in through sight; just one look at us and *they know.* How can we combat this negative attitude when teaching the content becomes routine for us?

The secret is to find a new method, idea, or tool to re-energize ourselves. We must become the source of positive energy! So many of those educators who took the first journey shared with me their successes with incorporating *Instant Teaching Tools for Health Care Educators* into their classes. Nursing faculty to in-facility staff educators at every level and corporate trainers have found a way to revitalize their educational presentations by traveling to their creative brain. This book is a short, do-it-yourself journey to a variety of destinations such as mandatory topics, curriculum and CE, and learning ideas for any content. It provides some detailed maps for you in your travel.

To ensure success, each of the 86 ideas has a preparation and implementation section to help you set up and follow steps to do the activity. There are symbols to make it easy to find the necessary information. Some pages are designed as ready to use, so you can simply copy and distribute them to your learners.

continued

Preface *continued*

I hope you smile as you read and use these instant teaching tools. How fun is a journey without some adventure and laughter? Enjoy them freely and generously as you begin your own personal road to teaching success. Only a real friend would share the secret to fun in learning; therefore, always explore new ways to teach that are fun and effective. It is the ultimate goal. Good luck and safe travel, friend!

—*Michele Deck*

Acknowledgements

Thank you to all the wonderful people who have made this book a reality. Thank you to each and every decision maker at Mosby. Thank you especially to Jackie and Jay Katz for their many productive years at Mosby. Every time I have the privilege to see the Katzs I am amazed at their creativity, their vision of the future of health care education, and their determination and commitment. I am so thankful that Mosby has chosen to make a second book like this a reality to assist all those in the field of health care education.

Thank you to Barb Watts, who is the most wonderful, kind, efficient, and tireless editor in the world. Her encouragement, patience, and attention to all details are what makes this book the useful tool it is to many. *More Instant Teaching Tools for Health Care Educators* and *Instant Teaching Tools For Health Care Educators* are a tribute to her excellent work! Thank you also to Ken Clark for being the best impromptu marketer in the world.

I would like to say a special thank you to some of my wonderful professional friends. Jeanne Silva is not only an enduring friend to me, but she is more than willing to answer the call for help morning, noon, and night. She taught me all about staff education, and she continues to teach me determination, loyalty, and to laugh. Nancy Hennen and Mandy Martin continue to amaze me with their growth and courage in pioneering new ideas in nursing. Thank you to Pam Brown-Stewart who is always willing to be a cheerleader and encourage me to try new ideas. A few years ago I met a special educator named Hal Vizinio, who has the most terrific creative gift. He was nice enough to share with me over the last few years. Hal, you are wonderful, and what you do is appreciated by many as a special gift from God.

Thanks a million to all of the spectacular professional colleagues of mine who unselfishly contributed ideas to this terrific collection. Thank you to Mary Beth, Sandra, Nancy, Sandy, Linda, Pam, Jeanne, Kathy, Sherry, Erin, Janet, Elaine, Lynn, Teresa, Jana, Mary Ann, Hal, Tom, Fran, Mary, Julie, Terry, Jeri, Susan, Chris, Bernie, Penny, and Ann. Your creativity is inspiring because it has the power to teach and transform when so much of our industry demands that! Special thanks to those who contributed not only to this book but to its predecessor. Thank you again to Mary Cahoon, Nancy Hennen, Mary LaBiche, Janet Fitts, and Jeanne Silva.

Thank you to the best friends anyone could have, Mary and Wayne LaBiche. Our life journeys parallel in only the most special of ways!

continued

Acknowledgements   *continued*

I would like to thank some very special teachers I have had, Bob Pike, Lynn Solem, Doug McCallum, Lori Backer, Jeanne Silva, and Heather Banton, who taught me to be a creative educator. I would like to thank my parents and sisters who have shaped the person I am today. I wish a long overdue thanks to Mary Ann Gruba, my eighth-grade teacher. She only taught me for one year, and I was very fortunate to have her. She taught me to write, which has proven to be an invaluable gift these many years later. Ms. Gruba, thank you!

Thank you to those of you who enjoyed *Instant Teaching Tools for Health Care Educators* so much that you have requested this continuation of new ideas. Thank you for the positive feedback and warm smiles as I have traveled. I feel blessed to have met you.

Last, but not least, thank you to my fun and fabulous husband, Brian, and our beautiful and understanding daughters, Brittany, Melanie, and Melissa, for their love and support. I know it's not always easy having a traveling mom. I love you always.

—Michele Deck

CONTENTS

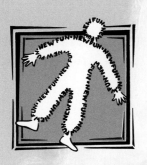

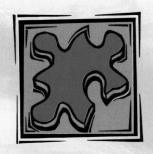

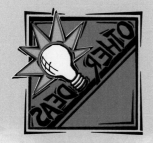

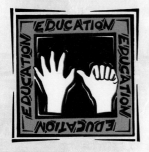

Contents *continued*

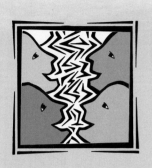

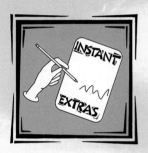

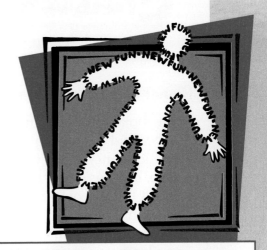

PART 1
CHALLENGES WE SHARE

CHALLENGES WE SHARE

Higher Numbers Of Assistive Personnel

As we look around in our healthcare facilities today we see a higher number and a variety of assistive personnel, all of them with educational needs just waiting to be satisfied. We must have quick, simple, and easy tools to use to teach the wide diversity of people. Some of those people may be intimidated by traditional-looking educational offerings that mimic school learning. Some of our assistive personnel may fall at various places on the literacy scale. These learners are new to those of us accustomed to teaching only professional people. They demand a fresh approach that is highly visual and interactive. The tools contained within this book offer information at a variety of levels of literacy. They can also be easily adapted to fit a variety of people in an assortment of healthcare settings, from schools of nursing and allied health fields to staff in a long term care facility (which has the most federally regulated mandated education requirements in any industry today, edging out even nuclear power plants). Many educators in healthcare facilities have been put in charge of the education of all personnel, because they have taught one group of healthcare personnel well. This can be overwhelming, and tools for use with varied groups are essential.

Limited Time

Why reinvent the wheel? Wouldn't it be nice to have a network of friends and other educators to share the ideas they have created and used with maximum effectiveness? This book is a collaboration of unselfish educators from a variety of clinical backgrounds and experiences that have used all of these ideas. They have been field tested in the toughest of all situations: with real healthcare personnel where time was always at a premium. This book has the white pages designed specifically to be copied and used immediately. This approach saves time in the development and preparation of educational offerings, whether live teaching sessions, or self-directed learning modules. Developing educational programs from scratch can take anywhere from 4 to 150 hours per one hour of content in the more complex lessons to be taught. Many educators say it takes them more time to teach others using high-involvement methods. They see their jobs as that of content delivery, not facilitator of what the participants actually learn. We must look to learning outcomes to know that we have done our jobs well and met our educator responsibilities. There is much more to teaching than just delivering content. The hard part is assuring yourself and others that learning has occurred in those who need it most.

Limited Resources

There are less people in exclusively education roles in healthcare facilities today. Most find the job of educator just one of the many jobs for which they are responsible. Many do not have support staff to type up exercises or do paperwork. There are many one person departments and large numbers of staff acting in teaching roles only a fraction of the time. These people need ready-to-use tools to instantly perform educational sessions. These tools can be used and adapted to a one-on-one to one-on-many format, whatever the case may be. There is less money available for buying teaching tools such as videos and prepackaged programs. Many are without budgets for simple items, such as binders and resource books or larger expenditures. Educators are looking for cheap and easy ideas to make their educational endeavors effective and their outcome focused. Some of these instant teaching tools require common props that are easily found or borrowed from home.

Results-Based Outcomes

Each of these instant teaching tools employs the most effective way to engage and focus the attention of learners today. Many of today's learners have been unconsciously conditioned by television to have very short attention and retention spans, which may vary from 7 to 20 minutes, and teaching without some learner feedback or involvement may be an effort in spinning our wheels. If our learners cannot recall the information we have imparted, how can they use it? How can we affect outcomes? How can information have an impact on patient care, processes, and procedures or systems if it does not reach the use or application phase? We invest in results and outcomes when we use high-involvement activities to impart information.

The population of our learners has changed over the last several years. Many of those we are teaching come to us to learn after a full, demanding life or a day spent working many hours. This presents the unique challenge of how best to teach learners who are mentally and physically fatigued in a learning setting. We do not want sleeping listeners. Those who are too fatigued to concentrate cannot remember information presented solely in lecture format. They require the high involvement these instant teaching tools provide.

High-Stress Environments

It's not unusual in this age of downsizing, right sizing, and frequent changes to find many of our learners performing their jobs under a high stress level. As stress and tension increases, learning retention decreases. Using these instant teaching tools can actually create a fun and relaxing learning environment, thereby increasing retention rates. Education today may be one of the few places it is safe to relax and step out of the usual role, whether for a short 10 minutes to a full semester of content. It is a time when we can enjoy the company of those we work with and actually experience a positive event that translates to team building. Yes, today many are working on healthcare teams, an ongoing relationship that sometimes suffers from the high-stress reaction of all or some members. These tools can bring a smile or even a laugh to be shared as a byproduct of active learning.

Familiar Formats

Many of these tools use familiar formats so that explanation time for activities is minimized. Notice the short time frame most of these instant teaching tools involve. This allows only a small time investment to use an idea. The simplicity of using tools such as crossword puzzles, quiz-type activities, boards, bingo sheets, and card activities reduces the time needed for explanation so maximum learning time is used. If any learning activity has an explanation to participants that takes more than about 5 minutes, it may be time to find another. Time is a premium in healthcare roles today, so getting into an activity as soon as possible is important.

Serious Content

Is it possible to teach the serious topics in healthcare in a fun way? Does it diminish the message? I have found that it is possible to teach any content in a way that is enjoyable to the learner. The process of learning can actually be joyful and engaging, not boring and dry. The seriousness of our jobs and the related information is not changed by these fun learning environments. Many find they are able to put the entangling emotions more easily to the side when they are highly involved in the learning process. Emotions and memories of difficult patient outcomes can interfere with the learning process and close learners to new information. The fun and lighthearted approach can move learners to a different set of emotions, those which are positive and newly energizing.

Repetition

High learning retention is built on frequent change, repetition, and involvement. Some learners think the responsibility they have when attending an educational session is to take up space in a chair. Have you met this person yet? They are expecting to receive the "Vulcan

Mind Meld." They expect us in one quick, easy step to transfer all of the knowledge and experience we have in our brains to them, to literally do a mind exchange. There is only one problem with this expectation. We are teaching humans, not Vulcans, and there is only one guaranteed way that humans learn. The key is involvement. Without it, there is little recall after 2 to 30 days of information presented once using lecture without involvement. These instant teaching tools can be used to deliver information or to review information in a highly involving way. This built-in involved repetition does not feel endlessly repetitive because different modes of learning are used.

Tradition

Many look to tradition to provide the most effective way to do something. Traditionally in healthcare education, lecture has been the most frequently used method to teach. Since this is what most educators are accustomed to doing, it is sometimes very comfortable for them to continue that same method. I'm reminded of a story about my family's holiday traditions. I traveled to Birmingham, Alabama, to spend the holidays with my sister, Mary Ann, who is an excellent chef. She has trained with Paul Prudhomme and maintained a catering business for many years. I watched her prepare a huge ham for baking, cutting about 4 inches off the shank area and setting it aside. I asked her what she was doing, and she said she could only use that portion as seasoning in her cooking at another time. I had never heard of this before, and asked her why.

She replied, "Mother always taught me to cut off this portion and put it aside. I'm not sure of the reason, but I'm sure its important to do it that way." I called my mother into the kitchen and asked her why she cut off the ham as she had taught Mary Ann. She said her mother had taught her to do that, but she had never asked why. On a later visit to my grandmother, I asked her why she always removed about 4 inches from the shank of the ham before baking it.

She said, "I didn't have a big enough baking pan in those days to bake the whole ham at once, so I cut off as much as necessary and used it as seasoning in beans and other dishes. Why do you ask?"

This cutting of the ham had become a family tradition, without anyone asking for a reason for the procedure. Sometimes I think this is the case with lecture-based teaching. Even though it is the hardest way for approximately 89% of average learners to learn, it maintains its high incidence of use. I think it is largely due to educator familiarity. Once another method of teaching presents itself for a possibility, most are just a little outside of their comfort zone trying it. After trying a new idea, there is less self doubt and more confidence built. This book provides a large choice of new teaching methods and tools for experimentation. No longer do we have to use traditional methods that we have found ineffective strictly because, "We've always done it that way!"

New Facilitator Roles

Some of the people who saw themselves in traditional educational roles in the past have found a gradual change or shifting of responsibilities to that of a facilitator. They are expected to perform in a human resource role, as well as the educator role. They are called on to work with teams, meet interpersonal and intrapersonal challenges, brainstorm and problem solve, as well as act in strategic planning. They are more an internal consultant than ever before, because of their highly tuned assessment and evaluation skills. Many have a broader background in patient care and health systems than any other person in their facility. I have also been amazed by the high number of healthcare professionals who can learn to do any job they face, accomplishing and excelling at it consistently. We are extremely adaptable creatures who harbor a secret knowledge base on how to be creative thinkers. Years ago the question might have been how do we make linen out of thin air; now it has grown to how do we create a new job or role that has an impact when all of our futures are so uncertain. We are talented and intelligent, and we value the assests of all who work with us and employ us.

The instant tools in this book can assist with the facilitator role some have adopted. It is just as important to create a positive human link among those in working relationships as it is to pass along content. Using these tools, both goals can be met simultaneously. What a great investment of time!

Building Memory

One of the components of building memory is outstandingness. The concept of outstandingness states that events and information that are outside the norm or unusual are easily recalled and remembered. This explains why it is easy to remember the unusual events and outcomes from patients and families of the past. In my years in labor and delivery nursing, the patients I recall are all the poor outcomes, not the happy and healthy mothers and babies I encountered. Does this sound familiar? One of the reasons these instant teaching tools help to build memory is that the approach to teaching is so different from the past history of learners. They may be used to years of the same old methods, and these are different and outstanding in comparison. This provides us with an additional memory advantage, in that the method itself assists in building recall.

Another retention-building concept employed in these tools is the chunking of content. Information is divided into manageable bits or bites for learner digestion, rather than in an overloading fashion. Chunking states that in short-term memory, humans remember seven plus or minus two items easily. Beyond that, recall becomes difficult. These tools employ refocusing elements that allow chunks of content to be remembered easily.

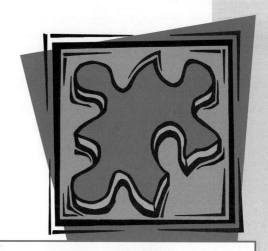

PART 2

INSTANT TOOLS FOR MANDATORIES

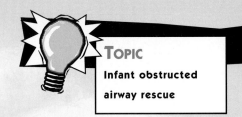

TOOL BOX

Doll or stuffed animal, toy slide, tiny doll, "happy 5th birthday" balloon, flapjack turner, plastic hand, service bell, spring-eyed gag glasses, object of obstruction such as a tiny ball, candy, penny, stuffed smiling face, Baby Heimlich Beat the Clock Steps sheet, Baby Heimlich Beat the Clock Box sheet, pens or pencils

BABY HEIMLICH BEAT THE CLOCK

Preparation

1. Obtain the following objects and maintain them in sequential order:
   (1) Doll or stuffed animal, the same size as an infant, that appears to be choking (popping eyes, open mouth, blue in color)
   (2) Toy slide and tiny doll to fit on the end of the slide—Tape the doll to the end of the slide face down with the head pointed downward.
   (3) "Happy 5th birthday" balloon—Blow up the balloon and tie it.
   (4) Flapjack turner.
   (5) Plastic hand.
   (6) Service bell with push-down button on the top.
   (7) Spring-eyed gag glasses.
   (8) Small ball, candy, penny, or any small object to demonstrate obstruction.
   (9) Stuffed smiling face.
2. Copy the Baby Heimlich Beat the Clock Steps sheet and Baby Heimlich answer key for each team, two to six participants per team, optimal.
3. Place the Baby Heimlich Beat the Clock Steps answer key in a large envelope, one per team.
4. Cut the Baby Heimlich Beat the Clock Steps sheet in strips, one step per strip, 13 strips total. (Note: There are four incorrect steps that will be left over when participants complete the exercise.)
5. Place the 13 strips into a small envelope, one envelope for each team.
6. Copy the Baby Heimlich Beat the Clock Box sheet, one for each participant.
7. Display the items on a table or area that offers easy access.
8. Provide a pen and pencil for each participant.

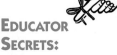

EDUCATOR SECRETS:

Participants review the content eight times in a quick format. Repetition increases retention of the learned material.

continued

By: Michele L. Deck, RN, MEd, BSN, ACCE-R

Baby Heimlich Beat the Clock *continued*

Option: Mark the back of all the strips in one set with the same alpha letter (i.e., set A, set B, set C, etc.). This prevents set mix up, if you plan to reuse the material.

Implementation

1. Divide participants into teams of two to six.

2. Recruit nine volunteers each to hold an object in front of the entire group.

3. Allow each volunteer to select an item from the display area.

4. Group together the volunteers holding objects 1 to 3 (1. doll, 2. slide, 3. balloon) and ask these volunteers to stand in number sequence in the front of the room to the extreme left of the audience (left to right: 1, 2, 3).

5. Group together the volunteers holding objects 4 to 6 (4. flap jack turner, 5. plastic hand, 6. service bell) and ask these volunteers to stand in number sequence in the center front of the audience.

6. Group together the volunteers holding objects 7 to 9 (7. spring-eyed gag glasses, 8. small object of obstruction, 9. stuffed smiling face) and ask these volunteers to stand in number sequence to the extreme right of the audience.

7. Explain life-saving measures in relation to the steps of infant obstructed airway rescue. Position yourself next to the group to the extreme left.

8. Ask volunteer number 1 to hold up the doll so all can see. Explain, "Step 1, identify infant choking. The infant begins to show signs of choking, difficulty breathing, turning blue, eyes show distress, mouth is open."

9. Ask volunteer number 2 to hold up the slide so all can see. Explain, "Step 2, slide the infant face down on your arm, with the head lower than the torso. Refer to the slide and the position of the doll."

continued

BABY HEIMLICH BEAT
THE CLOCK *continued*

10. Ask volunteer number 3 to hold up the "happy 5th birthday" balloon so all can see. Explain "Step 3, this "happy 5th birthday" balloon reminds us to give the infant five back blows between the shoulder blades."

11. Move to the middle group of volunteers and ask volunteer number 4 to hold up the flap jack turner for all to see. Explain, "Step 4, next we flip the infant over onto the other arm, with head lower than torso."

12. Ask volunteer number 5 to hold up the plastic hand for all to see. Explain, "Step 5, this reminds us of proper hand placement. Place the two middle fingers on the baby's sternum one finger's width below mid-nipple line."

13. Ask volunteer number 6 to hold up the service bell so all can see and ask the volunteer to press down on the bell five times. Explain, "Step 6, you need to press down on the infant's chest five times as deep as you press down on the bell."

14. Move to the group of volunteers at the far right. Ask volunteer number 7 to put on the spring-eyed glasses. Explain, "Step 7, look in the infant's mouth."

15. Ask volunteer number 8 to hold up the object selected to demonstrate obstruction. Explain, "Step 8, if you see the object, remove it."

16. Ask volunteer number 9 to hold up the happy face so all can see. Explain, "This represents a happy baby. Step 9, if the infant continues to choke, repeat the steps until the infant is no longer choking or becomes unconscious."

17. Ask each volunteer to take turns holding up their objects in order, so the learners can repeat each step in unison.

18. Ask the volunteers to scramble their order and have the group reorder them to their correct positions.

19. Have the volunteers return to their seats. Distribute a Baby Heimlich Beat the Clock Box sheet to each participant.

20. Ask participants to record in order the nine items that represent the steps on the Baby Heimlich Beat the Clock Box sheet without referring to the display area.

21. Have participants check their answers with the items displayed.

continued

12

BABY HEIMLICH BEAT THE CLOCK *continued*

22. Recruit one volunteer per team to act as a timekeeper and holder of the large envelope containing the Baby Heimlich Beat the Clock Steps answer key sheet. Supply a watch with a second hand or choose a participant that has a watch with a second hand. Do not reveal the contents of the envelope.

23. Distribute the small envelope with the cut strips of Baby Heimlich Beat the Clock Steps (one envelope per team).

24. Explain that on your signal each team works to place the Baby Heimlich Beat the Clock steps from the small envelope in correct order. Incorrect steps must be eliminated. When a team completes this task, they yell "Stop," and the team timekeeper records the time.

25. The team timekeeper opens the large envelope and removes the Baby Heimlich Beat the Clock Steps answer key. The team checks their performance for accuracy.

26. Give the team a second opportunity to race against the clock. The goal is to beat their first time while maintaining 100% accuracy.

BABY HEIMLICH BEAT THE CLOCK STEPS

Directions: Make a copy of this page for each team and cut the steps into strips.

Observe breathing difficulty in infant; cough is ineffective.	Slide infant face down over forearm with head lower than trunk.	Give five forceful blows between the shoulder blades with the heel of the hand.
Flip the baby over onto the other arm, with head lower than torso.	Place two to three fingers on the sternum, one finger's width below mid–nipple line.	Press down on the infant's chest five times; press as deep as you press down on the bell.
Look in the infant's mouth.	Remove foreign body, if visible.	Repeat these steps until the infant is not choking or becomes unconscious.
Slide the infant face down over forearm with head higher than trunk.	Press down on the infant's chest eight times; press as deep as you press down on the bell.	Help the infant on its back.
Give three back blows between the shoulder blades with the heel of the hand.		

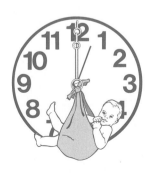

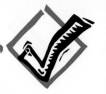

Baby Heimlich Beat the Clock Steps

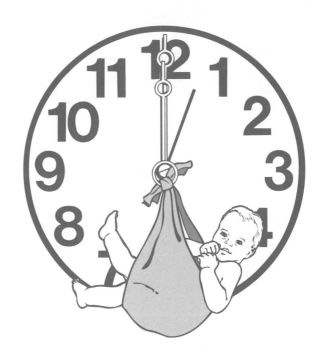

Answer Key

1. Observe breathing difficulty in infant; cough is ineffective.

2. Slide infant face down over forearm with head lower than trunk.

3. Give five forceful back blows between the shoulder blades with the heel of the hand.

4. Flip the baby over onto the other arm, with head lower than torso.

5. Place two to three fingers on the sternum, one finger's width below mid–nipple line.

6. Press down on the infant's chest five times; press as deep as you press down on the bell.

7. Look in the infant's mouth.

8. Remove foreign body, if visible.

9. Repeat these steps until the infant is not choking or becomes unconscious.

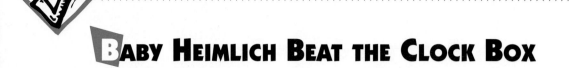

BABY HEIMLICH BEAT THE CLOCK BOX

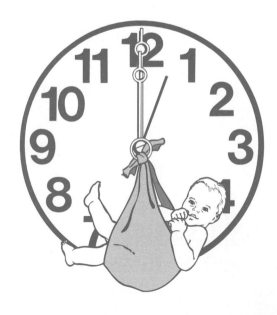

16

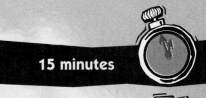

COMPETENCY MATCH

Preparation

1. Determine the number of participants and divide into teams (two to six participants per team). You will need Competency term and definition sets for each team.

2. Copy the Competency Match Terms (this is one set) and Definition Sheets (this is one set) and cut into strips. Keep sets separate.

3. Place one set of definitions and terms each in a separate envelope in random order.

Implementation

1. Establish teams of two to six participants.

2. Appoint or elect a leader for each team.

3. Distribute one envelope of definitions and one envelope of terms to each team leader.

4. Announce that each team will race to match up the competency terms with the competency definitions.

5. Ask the team leaders to empty the contents of each envelope in the middle of the table. Say, "Begin now!"

6. After team matching is complete, ask the groups to check their responses for accuracy.

7. Read the correct answers from the Competency Match Answer Key.

8. Allow time for discussion of why there was not 100% accuracy for each team. Point out the importance of competence when many have a different understanding of its components.

By: Pamela Brown Stewart, MN, RN, CCRN

TOOL BOX

Competency Match Terms sheet, Competency Match definitions sheet, Competency Match Answer Key sheet, colored paper (optional)

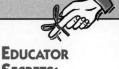

EDUCATOR SECRETS:

Print terms on one color of paper and definitions on another color for a visual distinction.

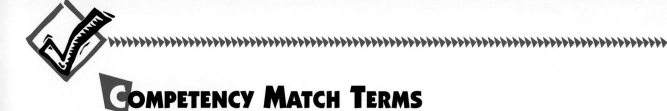

COMPETENCY MATCH TERMS

Directions: Copy this page and cut out each boxed term.

Standard

Competence

Competency

Continuing Education

Credentialing

Function

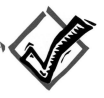

COMPETENCY MATCH DEFINITIONS

Directions: Copy this page and cut out each boxed definition.

> Possession of the knowledge, skills, and abilities necessary to fulfill the role functions of a designated setting.

> Actual performance in a designated setting consistent with established standards determined by the work setting.

> Provides current knowledge relevant to an individual's role responsibilities or field of practice.

> The process of granting authorization to provide specific care or services based on established criteria.

> A goal-directed, interrelated series of processes.

> An acceptable level of achievement or performance.

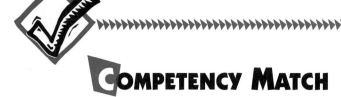

COMPETENCY MATCH

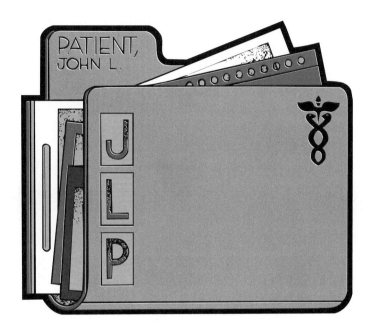

Answer Key

Competence

Possession of the knowledge, skills, and abilities necessary to fulfill the role functions of a designated setting.

Competency

Actual performance in a designated setting consistent with established standards determined by the work setting.

Continuing Education

Provides current knowledge relevant to an individual's role responsibilities or field of practice.

Credentialing

The process of granting authorization to provide specific care or services based on established criteria.

Function

A goal-directed, interrelated series of processes.

Standard

An acceptable level of achievement or performance.

TOPIC
Joint Commission on
Accreditation of
Healthcare
Organizations (JCAHO)
preparation

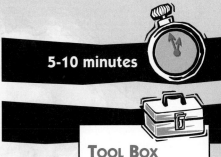

JCAHO Trivia

TOOL BOX
JCAHO Trivia
Questions and
Answers; buzzing
device or noisemaker;
watch or clock with
second hand; prizes

Preparation

1. Copy the JCAHO Trivia Questions and Answers.
2. Check current JCAHO standards to determine the desired response to JCAHO questions.
3. Create questions specific to the participants' organization. Include information to reflect what staff may need to know to prepare for their JCAHO survey.
4. Obtain a buzzer, whistle, or bell.

Variations

Copy JCAHO Trivia Questions and Answers onto an overhead transparency or onto flip chart paper.

Remember: If you use this method, reveal only one question at a time!

Implementation

1. Divide participants into teams of two to six.
2. Appoint or elect a leader for each team.
3. Give the leaders a response device (buzzer, whistle, bell).
4. Ask the leaders to test the response devices.
5. Announce that you will read a JCAHO Trivia Question and the first team to sound their response device will have five seconds to answer the question. If the team can't answer correctly within five seconds, another team can sound their response device and state the answer.
6. Start the game—read one JCAHO question at a time.
7. Monitor for the five second response time.
8. Discuss answer briefly.
9. Award points for each correct answer.
10. Award prizes based on highest number of points scored at the end of the round.

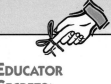

EDUCATOR
SECRETS:
Consider giving
everyone a prize for
participation.

By: Pamela Brown Stewart, MN,
RN, CCRN

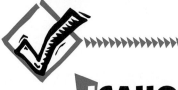

JCAHO Trivia

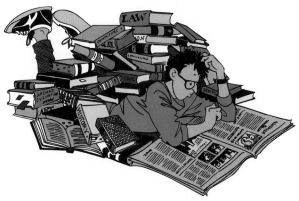

Questions and Answers

1. **True or false: The Joint Commission on Accreditation of Healthcare Organizations (JCAHO) is a federally funded agency.** (___1___ point)
   False. The JCAHO is a private, not-for-profit organization.

2. **How many hospitals and other healthcare agencies does the JCAHO accredit?** (___1___ point)
   JCAHO accredits more than 8,200 agencies (5,200 hospitals and more than 3,000 other organizations).

3. **What is the mission of JCHAO?** (___2___ points)
   JCAHO's mission is to improve the quality of care provided to the public. It was established in 1951 by the American College of Surgeons, the American College of Physicians, and the American Medical Association with the purpose of providing voluntary accreditation.

4. **How is the JCAHO accreditation achieved?** (___1___ point)
   Accreditation is achieved through an organization demonstrating compliance with standards that are developed collaboratively and published in documents such as the Accreditation Manual for Hospital (AMH).

5. **Name two reasons healthcare organizations seek JCAHO accreditation?** (___1.5___ points)
   It may be used to meet certain Medicare certification requirements.
   It enhances community confidence and reputation.
   It enhances medical staff recruitment.
   It expedites third-party payment.
   It often fulfills state licensure requirements.
   It may favorably influence liability insurance premiums.

6. **True or false: The standards found in the Management of Human Resources Section of the AMH is assigned to the Human Resources Department.** (___1___ point)
   False
   Add questions specific to your facility.
   Example:

7. **Where are copies of the JCAHO accreditation manuals located in your facility.** (___1.5___ points)

8. **Where is your organization's mission statement located?** (___2___ points)

9. _____

   _____

   _____

INFECTION CONTROL SHAPE UP!

Preparation

1. Copy Infection Control Questionnaire and Infection Control Shape Up sheets for each participant.

2. Copy Infection Control Shape Up Answer Key.

3. Obtain three different colored markers, crayons, or pencils for each participant.

Implementation

1. Distribute Infection Control Questionnaire; Infection Control Shape Up sheet; and colored markers, crayons, or pencils to each participant.

2. Ask participants to look at the top of Infection Control Questionnaire where it says "Color A, Color B, and Color C." Instruct participants to select a color for A, a color for B, and a color for C, and write the colors identified in the appropriate blanks. (See Infection Control Shape Up Answer Key.)

3. Have participants answer the questions on the Infection Control Questionnaire.

4. Ask participants to look at the Infection Control Shape Up sheet and match the numbered areas on the Infection Control Shape Up sheet with the corresponding question numbers on the Infection Control Questionnaire. Color the corresponding numbered area on the Infection Control Shape Up sheet with the color assigned to the answer's alpha letter. For example: A = Orange, B = Pink, C = Green.

5. Ask participants to identify the two important pieces of equipment used to help prevent the spread of infection that appear once the picture is colored in. (See the Answer Key—gloves and gown.)

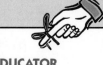

By: Sherry L. Blanchard, RN

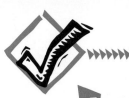

INFECTION CONTROL QUESTIONNAIRE

Color code your answers by writing in the colors selected for A, B, and C. Find the number on the "Shape Up" picture that corresponds to the question number, and color that area with the selected color for that alpha letter.

Color A _____

Color B _____

Color C _____

1. The single most effective way to prevent the spread of disease is:
   A. By staying home.
   B. Handwashing.
   C. Lining the trash cans.

2. Cross infections occur when:
   A. The infection is widespread throughout the body.
   B. A person is infected for the second time.
   C. An infection spreads from one person to another.

3. Reinfection occurs when:
   A. A person is infected a second time.
   B. Everyone in the unit gets infected.
   C. There is a respiratory infection.

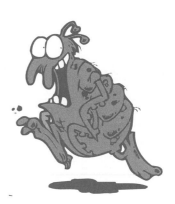

4. Linen that falls to the floor is considered:
   A. Contaminated.
   B. OK to use.
   C. A towel.

5. When washing your hands, it's important to:
   A. Stand close enough to the sink so your uniform touches.
   B. Use hand lotion.
   C. Clean under your fingernails.

6. Bacteria and viruses are:
   A. Always disease producing.
   B. Microorganisms.
   C. Always welcomed.

7. A patient is placed in isolation when:
   A. A patient is dangerous.
   B. The patient has a contagious disease.
   C. There is a shortage of rooms.

8. Sterilization is:
   A. Washing items with a disinfectant.
   B. The process of destroying all microorganisms.
   C. Only needed for surgery.

9. Disease can be spread by:
   A. Airborne contact.
   B. Direct contact.
   C. Both A and B.

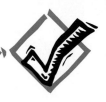

Infection Control Shape Up

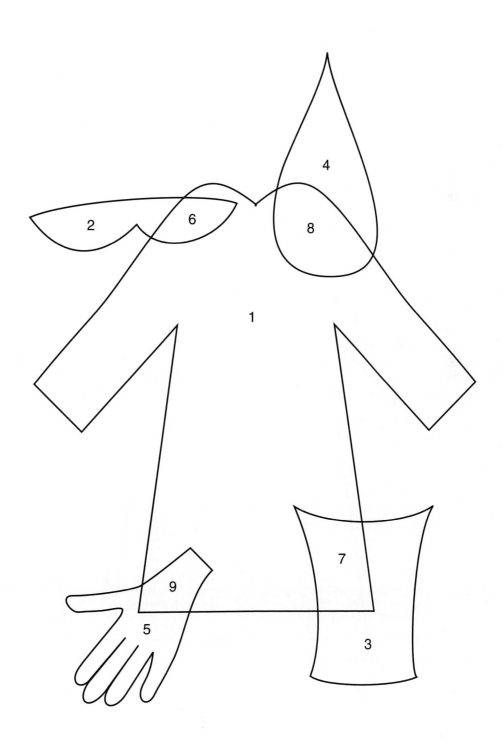

25

INFECTION CONTROL SHAPE UP

Answer Key

For example:

    Color A   Orange

    Color B   Pink

    Color C   Green

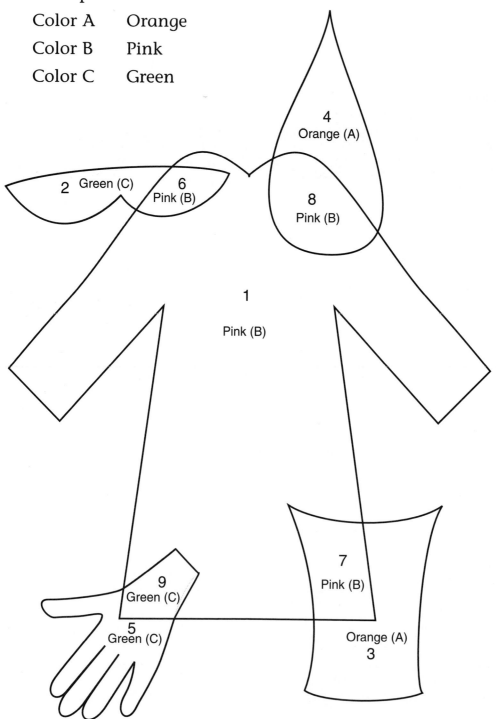

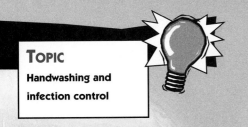

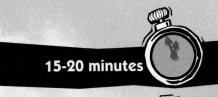

15-20 minutes

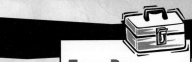

SINGING IN THE DRAIN

Preparation

1. Prepare the supplies for handwashing, such as soap and towels.

2. Obtain a watch or clock with a second hand.

3. Select a song to sing.

4. Start singing the selected song in your head. Use a watch or clock with a second hand to note when 15 seconds have passed. For example, a full chorus of *Jingle Bells* takes 15 seconds.

Implementation

1. Instruct the participants to sing the song in their heads through the timed portion as they wash their hands.

2. Invite the participants to practice the process so they can be sure of the full 15 seconds.

3. Explain that associating the timed segment of a song with hand washing will help them to be sure they have complied with the 15-second handwashing rule.

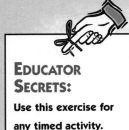

EDUCATOR SECRETS:

Use this exercise for any timed activity.

By: Erin E. Davis, MS, MEd, RRT

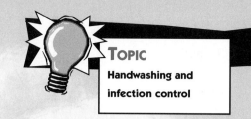

TOOL BOX

Watch or clock with a
second hand, sink with
running water, soap,
towels, ultraviolet
light, ultraviolet
illuminated powder
or lotion

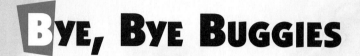

BYE, BYE BUGGIES

Preparation

1. Prepare the supplies for handwashing, such as soap and towels.
2. Obtain a watch or clock with a second hand.
3. Cover your hands with the ultraviolet powder or lotion
   (e.g., Glowgerm).

Implementation

1. Shake hands with all of the participants; place your left hand
   over their hand so that you are giving a two-handed shake.
2. Tell the participants that you will be discussing handwashing.
3. Ask participants to wash their hands normally. When they return,
   turn off the lights and illuminate their hands under an ultraviolet
   light to demonstrate the spread of germs. This demonstrates areas
   where germs remain after a normal handwashing.
4. Teach about proper handwashing.
5. Have the participants wash their hands for a full 15 seconds.
6. Illuminate their hands after proper washing to show
   improvement.

EDUCATOR SECRETS:

A visual demonstration
allows participants
to "see" the results
of something that
is normally only a
concept.

By: Erin E. Davis, MS, MEd, RRT
Mary N. LaBiche, MEd, RRT

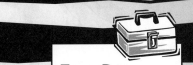

EMERGENCY DRUG QUESTIONS, NOT ANSWERS

TOOL BOX
Emergency Drug
Questions; Not
Answers First Round
and Second Round
Game Boards;
Emergency Drug
Questions, Not
Answers First Round
and Second Round
sheets; Emergency
Drug Questions, Not
Answers First Round
and Second Round
Answer Keys; buzzing
device or noisemaker;
Post-it™ notes; small
prizes or goodies

Preparation

1. Review Emergency Drug Questions, Not Answers First Round and Second Round sheets. If the information does not agree with policies and procedures of the learning facility edit the material to comply with the learning facility's policies and procedures.

2. Make an overhead transparency of the Emergency Drug Questions, Not Answers Game Board First Round and Second Round. (A poster/flip chart can be made instead, if desired.)

3. Make a copy of the Emergency Drug Questions, Not Answers First Round and Second Round sheets. Use these copies to read the answer when the team spokesperson picks a category and amount. The Answer Keys contain the correct questions that correspond to the category answers.

4. Obtain a buzzing device or noisemaker for each team to determine which team rings in first.

5. Collect small prizes or goodies (such as donuts, tootsie rolls, fruit snacks, pretzels, Post-it™ notes, etc.) to award to the participants at the end of the activity.

Implementation

1. Divide the group into two or more teams of three to six participants.

2. Appoint a spokesperson or leader for each team.

3. Pick a team to go first.

4. Display the Emergency Drug Questions, Not Answers First Round Game Board on an overhead transparency or flip chart.

continued

EDUCATOR SECRETS:
Equalize the competition, if possible. Learners find it more fun and less stressful when everyone has a turn to answer.

By: Janet Fitts, BSN, RN, CEN, TNS, EMT-P

EMERGENCY DRUG QUESTIONS, NOT ANSWERS *continued*

5. Place the buzzing device or noisemaker with the team spokesperson.

6. Provide the following directions:

   a. The spokesperson for the team selected to go first picks a category and an amount.

   b. The instructor reads the answer and amount for the selected category from the Emergency Drug Questions, Not Answers First Round sheet.

   c. A team may collaborate on their response for up to 5 seconds.

   d. The first team to buzz in has the opportunity to state the correct question.

   e. If the question stated is correct, the team is awarded the points attached to that question, as indicated on the game board.

   f. If the answer is incorrect, the other team(s) can answer, or you may choose to reveal the answer.

   g. After all answers are given, tally the points for each team. The team with the most points wins.

7. Use Post-it™ notes to cover categories and amount squares after they have been chosen. This makes it easy to see what has been eliminated.

8. Follow the same guidelines for the second round.

9. Award prizes to all participants.

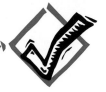

EMERGENCY DRUG QUESTIONS, NOT ANSWERS

First Round Game Board

Be Still My Heart	Heavy Breathing	It Hurts So Good	Gag Me, Man	Oh, Baby
1	1	1	1	1
2	2	2	2	2
3	3	3	3	3
4	4	4	4	4
5	5	5	5	5

EMERGENCY DRUG QUESTIONS, NOT ANSWERS

First Round

Be Still My Heart Cardiac Meds	Heavy Breathing Respiratory Meds	It Hurts So Good Analgesics	Gag Me, Man Antidotes	Oh, Baby Meds Used in OB Emergencies
1 Med given SL for chest pain.	1 First med in all respiratory emergencies.	1 Med given for chest pain, usually IV.	1 Med given for narcotic overdose.	1 Med given via infusion after delivery of placenta.
2 First med in symptomatic bradycardia.	2 Med usually given by nebulizer treatment at 2.5 mg per dose.	2 Narcotic that is good for orthopedic pain.	2 Med given to stimulate vomiting after overdose.	2 Med given in eclamptic seizures.
3 Med repeated every 3-5 min in cardiac arrest.	3 Med given SQ for anaphylaxis.	3 Nonnarcotic, nonsteroidal injectable analgesic.	3 Med that reverses benzodiazepine sedation.	3 Med that can stop premature labor.
4 First med for stable ventricular tachycardia.	4 Med given by IV loading dose, often followed by infusion.	4 Inhaled gas mixture self-administered for pain relief.	4 Ampule that is crushed and inhaled in cyanide poisoning.	4 Med used for eclamptic seizures when $MgSo_4$ is unavailable.
5 Med given for pulmonary edema in CHF.	5 Med given by metered dose inhaler at 0.65 mg.	5 Medication category for nonapproved controlled substances.	5 Naloxone 2 mg Thiamine 100 mg Dextrose 50% 25 g.	5 A potential uterine complication when giving oxytocin.

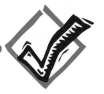

EMERGENCY DRUG QUESTIONS, NOT ANSWERS

First Round

Answer Key

Be Still My Heart Cardiac Meds	Heavy Breathing Respiratory Meds	It Hurts So Good Analgesics	Gag Me, Man Antidotes	Oh, Baby Meds Used in OB Emergencies
1 What is nitroglycerin?	1 What is oxygen?	1 What is morphine?	1 What is naloxone (Narcan)?	1 What is oxytocin (Pitocin)?
2 What is atropine?	2 What is Alupent (Proventil)?	2 What is meperidine (Demerol)?	2 What is syrup of ipecac?	2 What is magnesium sulfate?
3 What is epinephrine 1:10,000?	3 What is epinephrine 1:1,000?	3 What is ketorolac (Toradol)?	3 What is flumazenil (Romazicon)?	3 What is terbutaline (Brethine)?
4 What is lidocaine (Xylocaine)?	4 What is aminophylline?	4 What is nitrous oxide?	4 What is amyl nitrite?	4 What is diazepam (Valium)?
5 What is furosemide?	5 What is meta-proterenol?	5 What is Schedule I?	5 What is coma cocktail?	5 What is uterine rupture?

EMERGENCY DRUG QUESTIONS, NOT ANSWERS

Second Round Game Board

Twist and Shout	Grab Bag	Facts and Comparisons	Sock It To Me	What a Shock
1	1	1	1	1
2	2	2	2	2
3	3	3	3	3
4	4	4	4	4
5	5	5	5	5

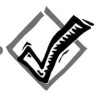

EMERGENCY DRUG QUESTIONS, NOT ANSWERS

Second Round

Twist and Shout Anxiolytics and Anticonvulsants	Grab Bag Anything Related To Pharmacology	Facts and Comparisons Drug Information	Sock It To Me Drug Administration	What a Shock Shock and Fluid Therapy
1 First med during tonic-clonic seizures.	1 "Fight or flight" system.	1 This book has information supplied by drug companies.	1 The most rapid route of drug administration.	1 Isotonic crystalloid most used in the field.
2 Med that also has cardiac uses.	2 Primary unit of solid measure in metric system.	2 One or more substances dissolved in water.	2 Most important piece of protective equipment.	2 Fluid of choice in hospital for hemorrhagic shock.
3 Med that can cause hyperactivity in children.	3 Must be administered through a filter.	3 Can be several of these names per drug.	3 Sodium bicarbonate deactivates this group of drugs.	3 A type of IV solution made up of proteins.
4 Calcium gluconate is the antidote.	4 The receptor that increases heart rate, force, and contractility.	4 The four major sources of drugs.	4 This can occur if IV tubing is not properly flushed before starting IV.	4 Common solution *not* indicated in fluid resuscitation.
5 IM drug for delirium tremens.	5 NAVEL.	5 BNDD, DEA, FDA, and FTC.	5 Name of this effect $NaHCO_3^- + CaCl^+$ $= NaCl + CaCO_3^\pm$	5 Volume expander derived from blood.

EMERGENCY DRUG QUESTIONS, NOT ANSWERS

Second Round

Answer Key

Twist and Shout Anxiolytics and Anticonvulsants	Grab Bag Anything Related To Pharmacology	Facts and Comparisons Drug Information	Sock It To Me Drug Administration	What a Shock Shock and Fluid Therapy
1 What is diazepam (Valium)?	1 What is sympathetic nervous system?	1 What is PDR?	1 What is intravenous?	1 What is normal saline?
2 What is phenytoin (Dilantin)?	2 What is gram?	2 What is a solution?	2 What are gloves?	2 What is blood?
3 What is phenobarbital?	3 What is mannitol?	3 What is trade name?	3 What are catecholamines?	3 What is colloid?
4 What is magnesium sulfate?	4 What is Beta-1?	4 What are animal, mineral, vegetable, and synthetic?	4 What is an air embolus?	4 What is D5W?
5 What is chlordiazepoxide (Librium)?	5 What are drugs that can be given ET: Narcan, atropine, Valium, epinephrine, and lidocaine?	5 What are agencies that enforce the narcotic control act of 1956?	5 What is H+ precipitation?	5 What is plasmanate?

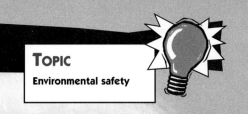

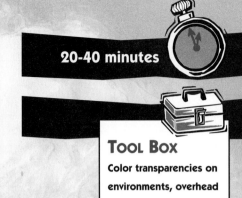

20-40 minutes

THE REAL PICTURE

TOOL BOX

Color transparencies on environments, overhead projector

Preparation

1. Take photographs of examples of unsafe environments, such as elderly patients' homes, poor work environments, and so forth.

2. Develop the photos and select those that clearly depict environmental safety hazards.

3. Turn the photos into color overheads.

4. Make sure that you have a complete set of overheads for each small group of two to five participants.

5. Mark one overhead in each set with a star to identify the special overhead that group will discuss for the entire class.

6. Make sure you have access to an overhead projector.

Implementation

1. Break your class into small groups of two to five participants.

2. Give each group a complete set of overheads.

3. Ask the participants to begin examining the overheads to see what is "right" or "wrong" with each one, paying particular attention to the one marked with the star.

4. Recruit a volunteer from each small group to come up front. This person places the transparency on the overhead projector and shows the entire group what their small group identified.

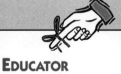

EDUCATOR SECRETS:

Color transparencies are a novel way to present information in small teams.

By: Elaine Frank
Lynn Lippitt

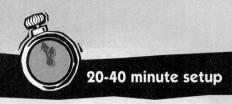

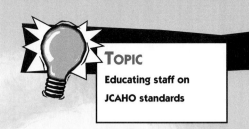

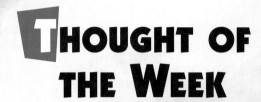

TOOL BOX

24″ × 36″ cork bulletin board for each unit or area, paint, coordinated colored paper, staff photographs, cartoons whenever possible, thought for the week about JCAHO issues

THOUGHT OF THE WEEK

Preparation

1. Decide which specific JCAHO topic to highlight on the bulletin board. This topic should address a general knowledge deficit among the staff. Select one thought for each week.

2. Take photos of the staff to include in your display.

3. After developing the photos, select those that best depict the information you are presenting.

4. Create brief text for the board display.

5. Paint the bulletin board an eye-catching color, such as orchid.

6. Develop a graphic to announce the topic.

7. Develop a standard layout for all offices to follow, and prepare the text to send out to each unit. Be sure to clarify the week it is to be displayed.

8. Use stationary headings such as *JCAHO Thought of the Week* and *Resources/Tools*.

9. Correlate JCAHO standards with your own organizational practice and requirements.

Implementation

1. Invite each unit to make the thought for the week the focus of discussion in each area in which it is posted. The thought for the week can be included in staff meetings, manager's meetings, and all educational offerings.

EDUCATOR SECRETS:

Add small candies or balloons to the boards. Use staff photos; it builds a sense of belonging.

By: Mary Cahoon, BS, RN

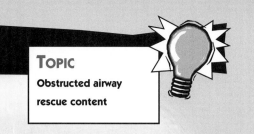

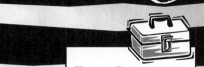

HEIMLICH QUESTIONS, NOT ANSWERS

TOOL BOX
Heimlich Questions,
Not Answers Game
Board on an overhead
transparency or poster;
Heimlich Questions,
Not Answers sheet and
Answer Key questions
sheet; buzzing device
or noisemakers;
Post-it™ notes; small
prizes or goodies

Preparation

1. Review the information on the Heimlich Questions, Not Answers sheet and answer key. If it does not agree with the facility's policies, procedures, and information, edit it appropriately.

2. Make an overhead transparency of the Heimlich Questions, Not Answers Game Board. (A poster can be made instead, if desired.)

3. Copy the Heimlich Questions, Not Answers. Use this copy to read the selected answer when the team spokesperson picks a category and amount.

4. Copy the Heimlich Questions, Not Answers Key to verify correct responses.

5. Obtain a buzzing device or noisemakers to determine which team rings in first.

6. Collect small prizes or goodies (such as donuts, tootsie rolls, fruit snacks, pretzels, Post-it™ notes, etc.) to award to the participants at the end of the activity.

Implementation

1. Divide the group into two or more teams of three to six participants.

2. Appoint a spokesperson or leader for each team.

3. Pick a team to go first.

4. Display the Heimlich Questions, Not Answers Game Board on an overhead transparency or flip chart.

5. Place the buzzing device or noisemaker with the team spokesperson.

continued

EDUCATOR SECRETS:
Equalize the competition, if possible. Learners find it more fun and less stressful when everyone has a turn to answer.

By: Jeanne R. Silva, BSN, RN, CCRN
Michele L. DECK, RN, MEd, BSN, ACCE-R

HEIMLICH QUESTIONS, NOT ANSWERS *continued*

6. Provide the following directions:

   a. The spokesperson for the team selected to go first picks a category and an amount.

   b. The instructor reads the answer and amount for the selected category from the Heimlich Questions, Not Answers sheet.

   c. A team may collaborate on their response for up to 5 seconds.

   d. The first team to buzz in has the opportunity to state the correct question.

   e. If the question stated is correct, the team is awarded the points attached to that question, as indicated on the game board.

   f. If the answer is incorrect, the other team(s) can answer, or you may choose to reveal the answer.

   g. After all answers are given, tally the points for each team. The team with the most points wins.

7. Use Post-it™ notes to cover categories and amount squares after they have been chosen. This makes it easy to see what has been eliminated.

8. Award prizes to all participants.

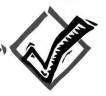

HEIMLICH QUESTIONS, NOT ANSWERS

Game Board

Step by Step	What If	Tell Me Why	Game Plan
1	1	1	1
2	2	2	2
3	3	3	3
4	4	4	4
5	5	5	5

HEIMLICH QUESTIONS, NOT ANSWERS

Step by Step	What If	Tell Me Why	Game Plan
1 This is asked before you perform the obstructed airway rescue.	**1** This is the phone number in your community to activate EMS.	**1** The question that you ask to make sure that the person is having a problem breathing.	**1** Of participants or instructors, games focus learning on this group of people.
2 A person looks like this when they are choking because they are not getting any air.	**2** When you are doing an obstructed airway rescue and the person spits out a piece of meat, you check this.	**2** This is why you say, "Are you choking?"	**2** This is what WII-FM stands for and is a universal motivator for learners.
3 You stand here to do the obstructed airway maneuver.	**3** When you ask a person that you think is choking, "Are you choking?" and they reply, "Yes, I am" you should do this.	**3** You continue to thrust until this happens.	**3** This activity is a review of this maneuver.
4 You put your thumb here when you're making a fist so that you don't harm the person.	**4** When a person who is choking leaves the room, you should do this.	**4** Pushing air back up forces whatever is blocking the throat to do this.	**4** The airway rescue maneuver is named after this person.
5 With your arms wrapped around the person, this is how you move your hands to push the air out.	**5** When a woman is nine months pregnant and choking, you should do this.	**5** One reason why your arms might not reach around someone.	**5** Using this activity fosters a sense of this.

Copyright © 1998 Mosby–Year Book, Inc.

HEIMLICH QUESTIONS, NOT ANSWERS

Answer Key

Step by Step	What If	Tell Me Why	Game Plan
1 What is "Are you choking?"	1 What is 911?	1 What is "Are you choking?"	1 Who are the participants?
2 What is a blue face, hand to throat, and leaning over?	2 What is "Are they breathing?"	2 What is to make sure they are having a problem breathing?	2 What is What's In It For Me?
3 What is stand behind the person?	3 What is do nothing?	3 What is the person spits it out or passes out (becomes unconscious)?	3 What is obstructed airway rescue or the Heimlich maneuver?
4 What is inside your fingers or fist?	4 What is follow them?	4 What is come up? (cough it up, spit it up)	4 Who is Doctor Heimlich?
5 What is upward?	5 What is chest compression and call for help?	5 What is obesity or pregnancy?	5 What is fun, knowledge, or competition?

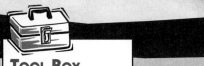

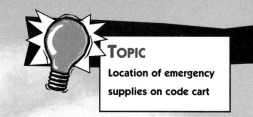
TOPIC
Location of emergency
supplies on code cart

TOOL BOX

Spin to Win wheel, word puzzle overhead transparency, poster, chalkboard or flip chart with easel, buzzing device or noisemakers, small prizes or goodies

SPIN TO WIN

Preparation

1. Copy the Spin to Win wheel, and follow directions.

2. Research where the emergency items listed below are located in the participant's facility and make a list. Use this list for your answer key.

   Emergency items:

   Laryngoscope

   Blades

   Lidocaine

   Epinephrine

   IV catheter

   Suction catheter

   1000 cc lactated ringer

   Guide wire

   Endotracheal tube

   Backboard

   Cut down tray

   Sterile gloves

   Sodium bicarbonate

   D50W

   Alcohol wipes

   McGill forceps

3. Obtain a buzzing device or noisemakers to determine which team rings in first.

4. Set up a flip chart and easel, chalkboard, or overhead for a mystery category word puzzle, such as *Defibrillate, Call Emergency Number,* or *Cardiopulmonary Resuscitation.* Leave a blank box or blank space visible for each letter in the puzzle.

continued

EDUCATOR SECRETS:

Play continues with more puzzles until all areas of the wheel have been discussed.

By: Jeanne R. Silva, BSN, RN, CCRN
Michele L. Deck, RN, MEd, BSN, ACCE-R

SPIN TO WIN *continued*

5. Display the Spin to Win wheel where it can be seen easily by the participants (on a wall or table).
6. Collect small candies for tokens (individually wrapped such as tootsie rolls).
7. Collect small prizes or goodies (such as donuts, tootsie rolls, fruit snacks, pretzels, Post-it™ notes, etc.) to award to the participants at the end of the activity.

Implementation

1. Divide the group into two or more teams of three to six participants.
2. Explain that the team in the control position (given the opportunity to answer the question) may collaborate on the answer for up to 5 seconds.
3. Tell the group in which category the puzzle fits. For example, "It is a thing."
4. Spin the arrow on the wheel. Be sure to spin and stop on all the areas.
5. When the spinner lands on an item, the team that buzzes in first controls the question.
6. A team representative gives the location of the item on which the spinner landed.
7. If the answer given is correct, the team receives a token or candy to hold.
8. The team giving the correct answer can pick a consonant to solve the mystery category puzzle, or can buy a vowel by turning in one previously earned token.
9. If the answer is incorrect, the instructor can give the other team a chance to answer the question or a chance to solve the puzzle.
10. If the team that answers correctly guesses a letter in the puzzle, they have up to five seconds to solve the puzzle.
11. Play continues until the puzzle is solved.
12. After all answers are given, the team with the most tokens wins.
13. Prizes can be awarded to all participants. Their knowledge has increased, and they are all winners.

SPIN TO WIN

Spinner

Directions:

1. Cut out the wheel, and paste it to a piece of cardboard.

2. Cut out the arrow, and paste it to a piece of cardboard.

3. Attach the arrow at the center of the wheel with a pivot clip.

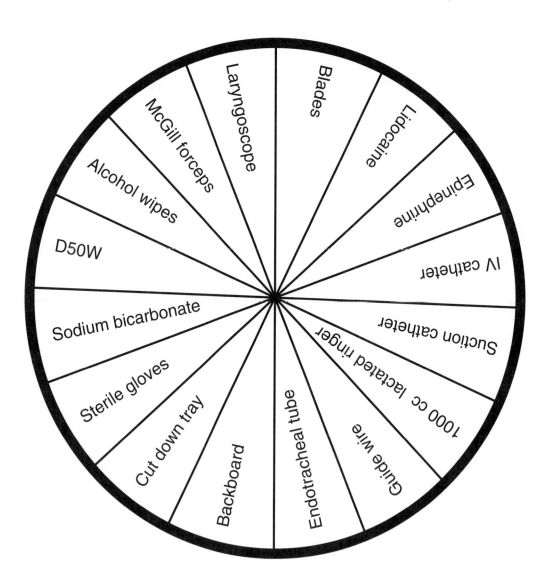

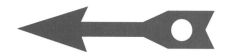

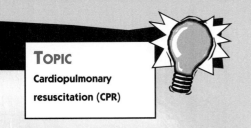

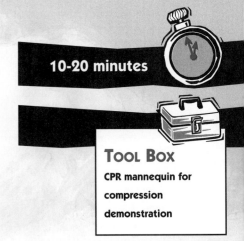

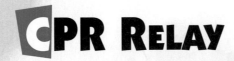

CPR Relay

TOOL BOX
CPR mannequin for
compression
demonstration

Preparation

1. Ready the mannequin for practice.
2. Clear space on the floor for relay.

Implementation

1. Divide the group into two or more teams of three to six
   participants.
2. Explain that each team will work together to complete all the steps
   of CPR *except* ventilations and compressions.
3. Ask each team to form a line.
4. Explain that when you say "Go," the following is to take place.

   a. The first member of each team lies on the floor to act as
      "victim."

   b. The second team member acts as "rescuer" and establishes
      unresponsiveness; calls for help; opens the airway; looks, listens,
      and feels; says "Two ventilations given"; and checks for a carotid
      pulse. The actual landmarks, head tilt, chin lift, and carotid
      pulse, must be found on the victim.

   c. Then the same second team member lies down to act as the
      "victim" and the third team member acts as "rescuer."

This round robin practice continues until the first victim gets a turn to
act as "rescuer."

5. Teams compete on accuracy of performance as they race a
   competing team to be the first to correctly finish their relay.
6. Use the mannequin for actual checkoff after this practice is
   complete.

**EDUCATOR
SECRETS:**
This assures that the
actual landmarks can be
found in a "real person"
victim.

By: Michele L. Deck, RN, MEd,
    BSN, ACCE-R

10-20 minutes

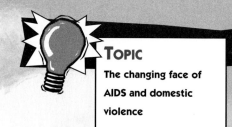

TOOL BOX

News Reels from the Front Questions, Not Answers Game Board on overhead transparency or poster; News Reels from the Front Questions, Not Answers questions sheet; News Reels from the Front Questions, Not Answers Answer Key; buzzing device or noisemakers; Post-it™ notes; small prizes or goodies

NEWS REELS FROM THE FRONT QUESTIONS, NOT ANSWERS

Preparation

1. Review the information on the News Reels from the Front Questions, Not Answers sheet and Answer Key. If it does not agree with the learning facility's policies, procedures, and information, edit it appropriately.

2. Make an overhead transparency of the News Reels from the Front Questions, Not Answers Game Board.

3. Copy the News Reels from the Front Questions, Not Answers sheet. Use this copy to read the appropriate answer when the team spokesperson picks a category and amount.

4. Copy the News Reels from the Front Questions, Not Answers Answer Key to verify correct responses.

5. Collect small prizes or goodies (such as donut, tootsie rolls, fruit snacks, pretzels, Post-it™ notes, etc.) to award to the participants at the end of the activity.

Implementation

1. Divide the group into two or more teams of three to six participants.

2. Appoint a spokesperson or leader for each team.

3. Pick a team to go first.

4. Display the News Reels from the Front Questions, Not Answers Game Board on an overhead transparency or flip chart.

5. Place the buzzing device or noisemaker with the team spokesperson.

EDUCATOR SECRETS:
Equalize the competition, if possible. Learners find it more fun and less stressful when everyone has a turn to answer.

NEWS REELS FROM THE FRONT QUESTIONS, NOT ANSWERS *continued*

6. Provide the following directions:

   a. The spokesperson for the team selected to go first picks a category and an amount.

   b. The instructor reads the answer and amount for the selected category from the News Reels from the Front Questions, Not Answers sheet.

   c. A team may collaborate on their response for up to 5 seconds.

   d. The first team to buzz in has the opportunity to state the correct question.

   e. If the question stated is correct, the team is awarded the points attached to that question, as indicated on the gameboard.

   f. If the answer is incorrect, the other team(s) can answer, or you may choose to reveal the answer.

   g. After all answers are given, tally the points for each team. The team with the most points wins.

7. Use Post-it™ notes to cover categories and amount squares after they have been chosen. This makes it easy to see what has been eliminated.

8. Award prizes to all participants.

News Reels from the Front Questions, Not Answers

Game Board

Positively Yours	Changing Times	Help Me	To Do List
1	1	1	1
2	2	2	2
3	3	3	3
4	4	4	4
5	5	5	5

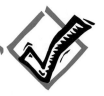

NEWS REELS FROM THE FRONT
QUESTIONS, NOT ANSWERS

Positively Yours	Changing Times	Help Me	To Do List
1 This is a sign or symptom of HIV.	1 The reported cases of HIV are increasing in this population.	1 This percentage of victims of domestic violence are women.	1 As healthcare professionals, we want to listen to victims of domestic violence in this way.
2 This is one way HIV is not transmitted.	2 This is the average cost of caring for one person with AIDS for one year.	2 This is the hotline number for the national coalition against domestic violence.	2 Some nurses are afraid to get involved with these patients because they think these matters are private.
3 This is one infection control procedure to prevent the spread of HIV.	3 According to the CDC these are three of the five states with the most reported AIDS cases.	3 This is the least likely phase for the victim to leave the perpetrator.	3 Domestic violence is misunderstood in part because of this myth.
4 This is one way HIV is transmitted.	4 One in 100 of this sex are HIV-positive in the United States.	4 The majority of these refuse to admit they have a problem.	4 This person may not want to leave the room during an examination of their partner.
5 You do not want to recap these to lower your risk of infection.	5 This drug is used as supportive treatment for HIV-positive patients.	5 This is the biggest danger the victim of domestic violence faces if she stays with the perpetrator.	5 This size of paper should be given to victims of domestic violence with referral phone numbers on it.

NEWS REELS FROM THE FRONT
QUESTIONS, NOT ANSWERS

Answer Key

Positively Yours	Changing Times	Help Me	To Do List
What is severe fatigue, sudden weight loss, fever, opportunistic infections?	Who are women, minorities, adolescents, babies, and people in rural areas?	What is 90% to 95%?	What is a caring and supportive way?
What is mosquito bites, animal bites, sharing toilets, sharing eating utensils, touching, hugging, nondeep kissing?	What is $38,300?	What is 800-799-7233?	Who are victims of domestic violence?
What is wash hands, wear gloves and protective clothing, minimize splashing, use sharp containers, one-way valves on masks, clean spills appropriately, specimen protocols?	What are Texas, California, New York, New Jersey, Florida?	What is the loving reconciliation phase?	What is romance?
What is exposure to blood products; sexual transmission; prenatal, perinatal, postnatal infection?	Who are men?	Who are perpetrators of domestic violence?	Who is the perpetrator of domestic violence?
What are needles?	What is AZT or antiviral drugs?	What is her death?	What is small or card sized?

RESCUE QUESTIONS, NOT ANSWERS

Preparation

1. Review the information on the Rescue Questions, Not Answers sheet and Rescue Questions, Not Answers Answer Key. If it does not agree with the learning facility's policies, procedures, and information, edit it appropriately.

2. Make an overhead transparency of the Rescue Questions, Not Answers Game Board.

3. Copy the Rescue Questions, Not Answers sheet. Use this copy to read the appropriate answer when the team spokesperson picks a category and amount.

4. Copy the Rescue Questions, Not Answers Answer Key as a reference to verify correct responses.

5. Collect small prizes or goodies (food such as donuts, tootsie rolls, fruit snacks, pretzels; Post-it™ notes; etc.) to award to the participants at the end of the activity.

Implementation

1. Divide the group into two or more teams of three to six participants.

2. Appoint a spokesperson or leader for each team.

3. Pick a team to go first.

4. Display the Rescue Questions, Not Answers Game Board on an overhead transparency or flip chart.

5. Place the buzzing device or noisemaker with the team spokesperson.

continued

By: Jeanne R. Silva, BSN, RN, CCRN

TOOL BOX
Rescue Questions, Not Answers Game Board on overhead transparency or poster; Rescue Questions, Not Answers questions sheet; Rescue Questions, Not Answers Answer Key; buzzing device or noisemakers; Post-it™ notes; small prizes or goodies

EDUCATOR SECRETS:
Equalize the competition, if possible. Learners find it more fun and less stressful when everyone has a turn to answer.

RESCUE QUESTIONS, NOT ANSWERS *continued*

6. Provide the following directions:

   a. The spokesperson for the team selected to go first picks a category and an amount.

   b. The instructor reads the answer and amount for the selected category from the Rescue Questions, Not Answers sheet.

   c. A team may collaborate on their response for up to five seconds.

   d. The first team to buzz in has the opportunity to state the correct question.

   e. If the question stated is correct, the team is awarded the points attached to that question, as indicated on the game board.

   f. If the answer is incorrect, the other team(s) can answer, or you may choose to reveal the answer.

   g. After all answers are given, tally the points for each team. The team with the most points wins.

7. Use Post-it™ notes to cover categories and amount squares after they have been chosen. This makes it easy to see what has been selected.

8. Award prizes to all participants.

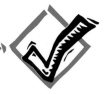

RESCUE QUESTIONS, NOT ANSWERS

Game Board

What's My Name	Give It To Me	A Little or A Lot	All Mixed Up	Watch and See
1	1	1	1	1
2	2	2	2	2
3	3	3	3	3
4	4	4	4	4
5	5	5	5	5

RESCUE QUESTIONS, NOT ANSWERS

What's My Name	Give It To Me	A Little or A Lot	All Mixed Up	Watch and See
1 — This drug increases blood pressure and increases urine output in low doses.	1 — This drug increases heart rate and is supplied in 1 mg Bristojet.	1 — This drug increases blood pressure 1-2 mg is low dose 3-10 mg is medium dose >10 mg is high dose.	1 — This drug increases heart rate and urine output 200 mg/250 cc.	1 — This drug increases urine output in low doses and increases blood pressure.
2 — This drug increases heart rate.	2 — This drug increases blood pressure and is supplied in 200 mg vials or ampules.	2 — This drug increases heart rate .5-1.0 mg 2 mg maximum.	2 — This drug increases blood pressure 4 mg/250 cc.	2 — Diuretic used for fluid overload.
3 — This drug is used to correct acidosis.	3 — This drug increases blood pressure and is supplied in 1 mg vials or ampules.	3 — This drug suppresses ventricular arrhythmias 1-1.5 mg/kg every 5-10 min.	3 — This drug is given for arrhythmias 2 gm/500 cc 1-4 mg/min.	3 — This drug decreases ventricular arrhythmias.
4 — This drug is used to control arrhythmias.	4 — This drug is given for ventricular arrhythmias and is supplied in 100 mg Bristojet.	4 — This drug increases heart rate 1 mg of 1:100,000 every 3-5 min.	4 — This drug increases heart rate 1 mg/250 cc.	4 — This drug corrects acidosis.
5 — This drug is a potent vasoconstrictor used to increase blood pressure.	5 — This drug is given for complete heart block, especially in heart transplant patients, supplied in 1 mg ampule or vial.	5 — Give 1 mg/kg of this drug, then check ABGs.	5 — This drug decreases blood pressure and preload used in MI patients 50 mg/250 cc.	5 — This drug increases blood pressure and decreases urine output.

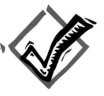

RESCUE QUESTIONS, NOT ANSWERS

Answer Key

What's My Name	Give It To Me	A Little or A Lot	All Mixed Up	Watch and See
1 What is dopamine?	1 What is atropine or epinephrine?	1 What is dopamine?	1 What is dopamine?	1 What is dopamine?
2 What is atropine, epinephrine, or Isuprel?	2 What is dopamine?	2 What is atropine?	2 What is Levophed?	2 What is Lasix?
3 What is sodium bicarbonate?	3 What is Levophed?	3 What is lidocaine?	3 What is lidocaine?	3 What is lidocaine, Pronestyl, bretyliem, or amiodarone?
4 What is lidocaine, Pronestyl, bretylium, or amiodarone?	4 What is lidocaine?	4 What is epinephrine?	4 What is Isuprel?	4 What is sodium bicarbonate?
5 What is Levophed, or norepinephrine?	5 What is Isuprel?	5 What is sodium bicarbonate?	5 What is Tridil?	5 What is Levophed?

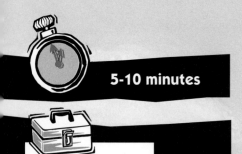
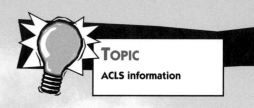
TOOL BOX

ACLS Commandments

THE ACLS COMMANDMENTS

Preparation

1. Copy one ACLS Commandments sheet for each participant.

Implementation

1. Distribute ACLS Commandments to each participant.
2. Read each Commandment aloud.
3. Point out key content as participants chuckle.

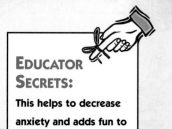

EDUCATOR SECRETS:

This helps to decrease anxiety and adds fun to your class.

By: Ann Eubanks, RN, CCRN
Tom Wilson
Fran Kelly

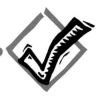

THE ACLS COMMANDMENTS

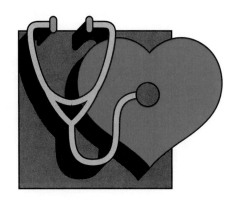

1. Thou shalt honor thy primary survey.

2. Thou shalt not defibrillate any person other than the one in ventricular fibrillation, unless they are severely depressed!

3. Thou shalt not ever defibrillate thy patient without first checking for a pulse.

4. Honor both thy compressions AND ventilations.

5. Thou shalt consider all possible causes of pulseless electrical activity.

6. Thou shalt always check two leads when asystole appears on the monitor. (The patient could be in the bathroom!)

7. Thou shalt always consider saying, "Get the transcutaneous pacemaker," before using atropine in the bradycardia algorithm.

8. Honor thy patient who complains of chest pain.

9. Thou shalt remember to give oxygen to an acute MI patient, or thou shalt surely have to test over and over again until you do.

10. Thou shalt honor thy instructors with bribery, or any other methods you can think of . . .

11. Thou shalt not administer lidocaine to a bradycardic patient with PVCs, lest they will surely die, and thou shalt get another algorithm to manage.

12. Thou shalt always assume wide-complex tachycardia is v-tach until proven otherwise by at least two experienced cardiologists.

13. Thou shalt heed the voices coming forth from within the automated external defibrillator.

14. CPR, CPR, CPR, CPR, CPR, and CPR!!!

15. Thou shalt remember "stacked shocks" do not describe the trucks seen at a monster truck rally.

16. Thou shalt consider withholding thrombolytics in the presence of bleeding hemorrhoids.

5-20 minutes

TOOL BOX

**Know Your Fire
Extinguishers Crossword
Puzzle, Know Your Fire
Extinguishers Answer
Key, pens or pencils**

KNOW YOUR FIRE EXTINGUISHERS CROSSWORD PUZZLE

Preparation

1. Copy Know Your Fire Extinguishers Crossword Puzzle for each participant. Use this as an introduction to the lesson or as a review after the lesson.

2. Copy Know Your Fire Extinguishers Answer Key.

3. Provide pens or pencils.

Variation

1. Use a poster printer copy machine to turn the crossword into a poster-size image.

2. Plan for groups of two to six to discuss and fill in the poster-size copy of the crossword puzzle before or after your lesson.

Implementation

1. Distribute a Know Your Fire Extinguishers Crossword Puzzle to each participant.

2. Challenge your learners to complete the puzzle as individuals or as teams.

3. Share the correct answers as you desire.

4. The puzzle may also be sent out to reinforce learning days or weeks after the lesson.

EDUCATOR SECRETS:

**If you have different
ability levels in your
session, pair learners of
opposite abilities to
maximize benefits
to all.**

By: Michele L. Deck, RN, MEd, BSN, ACCE-R

60

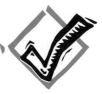

KNOW YOUR FIRE EXTINGUISHERS

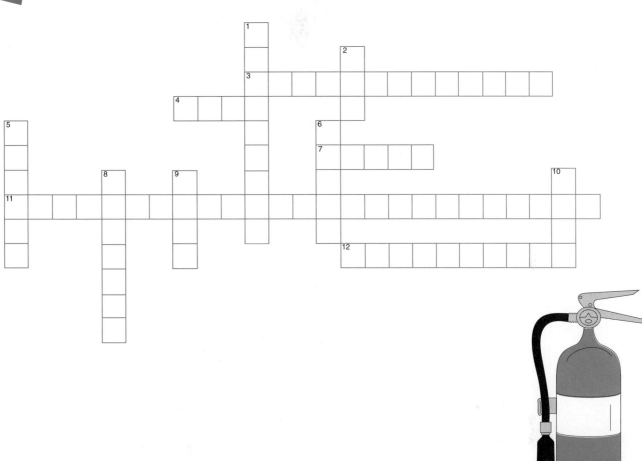

Across

3. To obtain the proper extinguisher for a trash can fire, you must open the cabinet door labeled _____ _____.

4. Using either type of extinguisher to put out a fire, you must direct the nozzle at the _____ of the fire.

7. This is what the *A* in RACE represents.

11. Type of fire extinguisher used to put out a fire caused by sparking cord and plugged to a pump.

12. The CO_2 extinguisher puts out _____ fires.

Down

1. Both types of fire extinguishers have a _____ _____ in the handle, which needs to be pulled before use.

2. CO_2 extinguishers are usually this color.

5. This is what the *R* in RACE process represents.

6. A trash can fire is extinguished using a _____ extinguisher.

8. This step proceeds *extinguish* in the RACE response.

9. _____ extinguishers are located on every wing of a nursing unit.

10. Before entering a room to extinguish a fire, you must _____ the closed door with the back of your hand.

61

KNOW YOUR FIRE EXTINGUISHERS

Answer Key

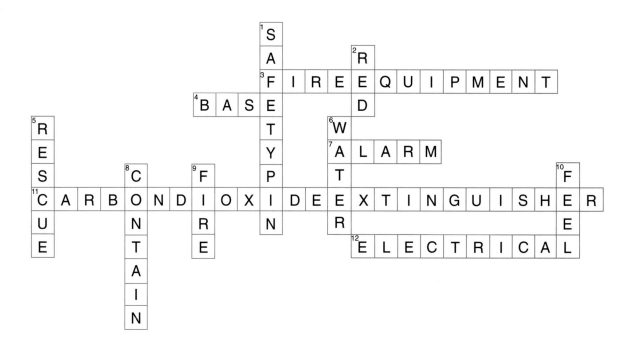

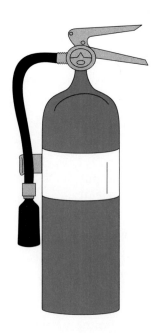

Across

3. Fire equipment
4. Base
7. Alarm
11. Carbon dioxide extinguisher
12. Electrical

Down

1. Safety pin
2. Red
5. Rescue
6. Water
8. Contain
9. Fire
10. Feel

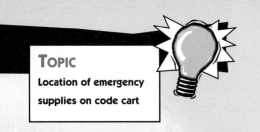

TOPIC
Location of emergency
supplies on code cart

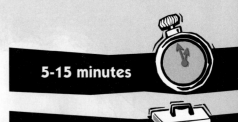
WHERE IS IT?

Preparation

1. Review all Where Is It? information to make sure it agrees with the learning facility's policies and procedures.

2. Copy the Where Is It? question sheet for each participant.

3. Complete the Where Is It? Fill-In diagram with the contents of the learning facility's code cart and make a copy for each participant. (See example on pp. 67-68.)

4. Complete a copy of the Where Is It? questions and keep it for your answer key.

5. Make sure all participants have a pen or pencil.

Implementation

1. Distribute the Where Is It? question sheet and the completed Where Is It? Fill-In diagram sheets to each participant.

2. Challenge participants to complete the Where Is It? question sheet using the completed Where Is It? diagram as a guide, individually or as a team.

3. Share the correct answers as you desire.

Note: The completed Where Is It? question sheet and completed Where Is It? diagram may also be sent out to reinforce learning days or weeks after the lesson.

By: Michele L. Deck, RN, MEd,
    BSN, ACCE-R
    Jeanne R. Silva, BSN,
    RN, CCRN

EDUCATOR
SECRETS:
This is a fun way to
learn and remind where
emergency supplies are
located.

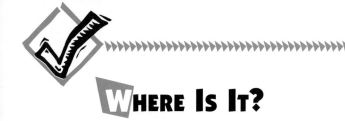

WHERE IS IT?

Questions

1. You need to start an IV. Where are the needed supplies to accomplish this?

Supplies	Location
Alcohol/betadine preps	_____
Tourniquets	_____
IV catheter	_____
IV tubing	_____
Tape	_____
Gauze	_____
IV dressing	_____
Fluid	_____

2. The patient needs to be connected to the defibrillator and defibrillated. Find what you need to get this done. (Assume the machine is out of paper.)

Supplies	Location
EKG leads	_____
Alcohol preps	_____
EKG paper	_____
Defibrillation pads and gel	_____

3. The patient needs the following drug therapy. Where is everything?

Supplies	Location
Atropine	_____
Epinephrine	_____
Lidocaine	_____
Isuprel for infusion	_____
Dopamine for infusion	_____
Ivac tubing	_____
2 gms xylocaine in 500 cc D5W	_____

4. Your patient is going to be intubated. Get what you need.

Supplies	Location
Endotracheal tube	_____
Lubricant	_____
Tape	_____
Benzion	_____
10-cc syringe	_____
Suction catheter	_____
Yankauer suction catheter	_____
Foot pump	_____

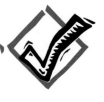

WHERE IS IT?

Fill-In

Drawer 1

Drawer 2

Drawer 3

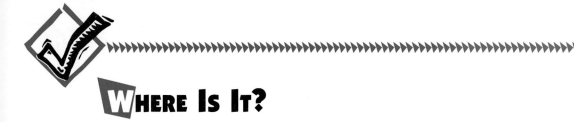
Fill-In

Drawer 4

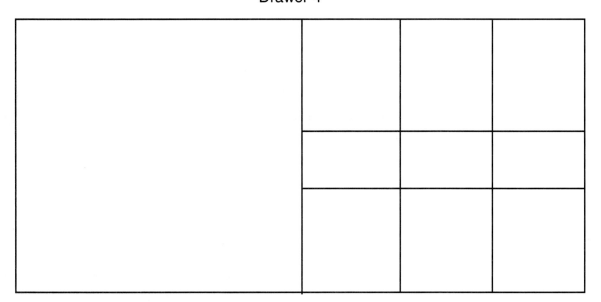

Bottom of cart

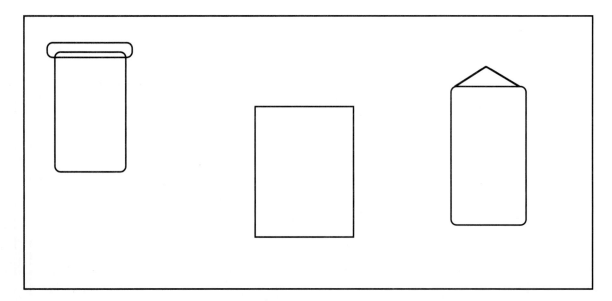

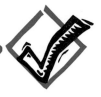

WHERE IS IT?

Fill-In Sample Answer Key

Drawer 1

Blood pressure cuff / Stethescope	Defibrillation creme	Medication
Xylocaine ointment / Leads		
Larnygoscopes Blades / Lubricant		

Drawer 2

Isuprel	Pronestyl		22-gauge needles	Syringes
Dopamine	Pronestyl		21-gauge needles	Syringes
Dobutamine	Lasix	Verapamil	18-gauge needles	Syringes
Bretylium	Lasix	NaCl	Betadine preps / Alcohol preps	Premixed lidocaine / Microdrip tubing

Drawer 3

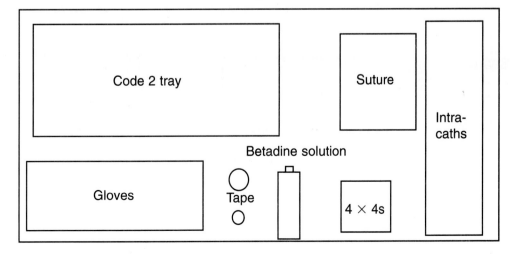

Code 2 tray

Suture

Intra-caths

Betadine solution

Gloves

Tape

4 × 4s

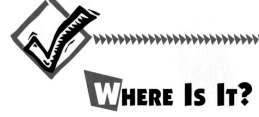

WHERE IS IT?

Fill-In Sample Answer Key

Drawer 4

Blood Administration Set	Microdrip Tubing	Volume Infusion Set	Extension Tubing Intracath
	Tourniquet	Tape	Med Label
Fluids	IV Catheters	IV Catheters	IV Catheters

Bottom of cart

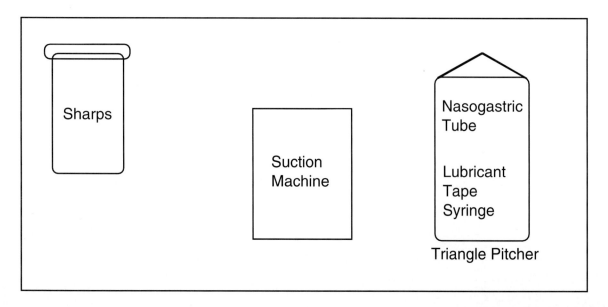

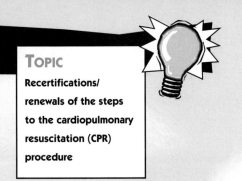
TOPIC

Recertifications/
renewals of the steps
to the cardiopulmonary
resuscitation (CPR)
procedure

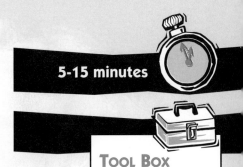

ROUND ROBIN CPR

TOOL BOX

CPR procedure
(for example, American
Red Cross To Save a
Life), CPR mannequin

Preparation

1. Review the CPR procedure to make sure you are familiar with it.
2. Obtain a CPR mannequin.

Implementation

1. Ask participants to form a circle around the CPR mannequin.
2. Explain that participants will take turns to state a CPR step and demonstrate the appropriate action.
3. Pick someone in the circle to go first.
   a. The first participant steps up to the mannequin and says, "Establish unresponsiveness," while demonstrating the action.
   b. The next participant to the right steps up and says step two; "Call for help."
   c. Participant number three steps up and says, "Open the airway," and demonstrates the required action.
4. Continue around the circle until the CPR procedure is complete. If anyone needs assistance, the group can offer hints for the correct step in the process.

EDUCATOR SECRETS:

This is a fun way to
review emergency
processes with the
support of peers.

By: Michele L. Deck, RN, MEd,
BSN, ACCE-R

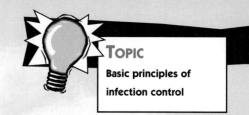

TOOL BOX

Infection Control with a Smile sheet, Infection Control with a Smile Answer Key, pens or pencils

INFECTION CONTROL WITH A SMILE

Preparation

1. Copy Infection Control with a Smile sheet for each participant.
2. Copy the Infection Control with a Smile Answer Key.
3. Provide a pen or pencil for each participant.

Implementation

1. Distribute Infection Control with a Smile to each participant.
2. Make sure everyone has a pen or pencil.
3. Ask the participants to complete the multiple-choice questions.
4. Read aloud the correct answers.

EDUCATOR SECRETS:

Smile when you read the answers. Provide the Infection Control with a Smile Answer Key as a handout to reinforce learned information.

By: Hal Vizino

70

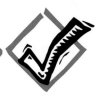

INFECTION CONTROL WITH A SMILE

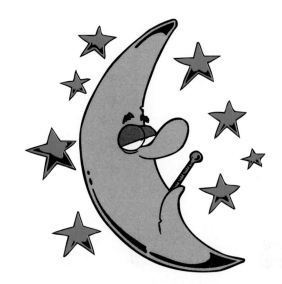

Directions: Circle the correct answers.

1. What is a nosocomial infection?

    a. One that is hospital acquired.

    b. One that has no socoms.

    c. One that has to do with the nose.

    d. One that is socially acquired.

2. Two sources of infection in the hospital environment include:

    a. Candy and pop.

    b. Computers and the gift shop.

    c. Trash and patient rooms.

    d. Information desk and AV media.

3. Which one is *not* a major vehicle for infection:

    a. Food.

    b. Water.

    c. Limousine.

    d. Drugs.

4. Three links in the "chain of infection" include:

    a. Means/Hostess/Source.

    b. Host/Source/Car (means of transportation).

    c. Host/Means/Cedar Point (point of origin).

    d. Source/Means/Host.

5. Which one of the following is *not* a type of patient who is more susceptible to infection?

    a. Diabetic.

    b. Cartoon character.

    c. Elderly.

    d. Newborn.

INFECTION CONTROL WITH A SMILE

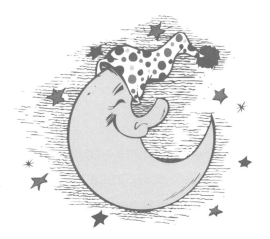

6. The most important means to prevent the spread of infection is:

    a. Showering twice a day.

    b. Handwashing.

    c. Ironing your shirts and blouses.

    d. Polishing your shoes.

7. Check the following five times in a workday when handwashing should be done.

    _____ Before reading a magazine.

    _____ After handling contaminated articles.

    _____ After patient contact.

    _____ After chewing gum.

    _____ After use of the bathroom.

    _____ Before going home.

    _____ Before invasive procedures.

8. Handwashing techniques. True (T) or false (F).

    _____ Comb your hair after drying your hands.

    _____ Turn off the faucet before drying your hands.

    _____ Clean under your nails.

    _____ Take rings and jewelry off before washing.

    _____ Thoroughly rinse hands and wrists.

    _____ Apply friction to all surfaces for at least 10 seconds.

    _____ Wash your forearms and face with your hands.

    _____ Wet your comb with your hand, then comb your hair.

    _____ Work up a lather.

    _____ Skip handwashing after using the restroom.

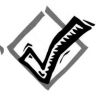

INFECTION CONTROL WITH A SMILE

Answer Key

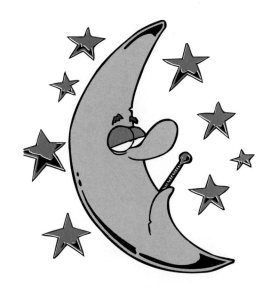

1. What is a nosocomial infection?

    ✔ a. One that is hospital acquired.

    b. One that has no socoms.

    c. One that has to do with the nose.

    d. One that is socially acquired.

2. Two sources of infection in the hospital environment include:

    a. Candy and pop.

    b. Computers and the gift shop.

    ✔ c. Trash and patient rooms.

    d. Information desk and AV media.

3. Which one is *not* a major vehicle for infection:

    a. Food.

    b. Water.

    ✔ c. Limousine.

    d. Drugs.

4. Three links in the "chain of infection" include:

    a. Means/Hostess/Source.

    b. Host/Source/Car (means of transportation).

    c. Host/Means/Cedar Point (point of origin).

    ✔ d. Source/Means/Host.

5. Which one of the following is *not* a type of patient who is more susceptible to infection?

    a. Diabetic.

    ✔ b. Cartoon character.

    c. Elderly.

    d. Newborn.

INFECTION CONTROL WITH A SMILE

Answer Key

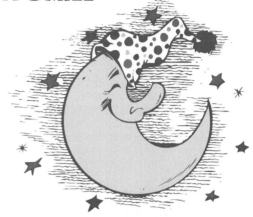

6. The most important means to prevent the spread of infection is:

   a. Showering twice a day.

   ✔ b. Handwashing.

   c. Ironing your shirts and blouses.

   d. Polishing your shoes.

7. Check the following five times in a workday when handwashing should be done.

   _____ Before reading a magazine.

   ___✔___ After handling contaminated articles.

   ___✔___ After patient contact.

   _____ After chewing gum.

   ___✔___ After use of the bathroom.

   ___✔___ Before going home.

   ___✔___ Before invasive procedures.

8. Handwashing techniques. True (T) or false (F).

   ___F___ Comb your hair after drying your hands.

   ___F___ Turn off the faucet before drying your hands.

   ___T___ Clean under your nails.

   ___T___ Take rings and jewelry off before washing.

   ___T___ Thoroughly rinse hands and wrists.

   ___T___ Apply friction to all surfaces for at least 10 seconds.

   ___F___ Wash your forearms and face with your hands.

   ___F___ Wet your comb with your hand, then comb your hair.

   ___T___ Work up a lather.

   ___F___ Skip handwashing after using the restroom.

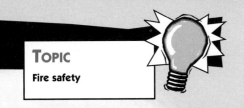

5-10 minutes

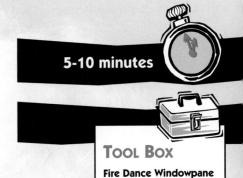

TOOL BOX
Fire Dance Windowpane
sheet, music, audio
equipment

THE FIRE DANCE

Preparation

1. Copy the Fire Dance Windowpane for each participant.

2. Review the four-step fire code:

   P—Patient or personnel out

   P—Pull the alarm

   D—Dial _____ (Add the facility's emergency number; for example, 33)

   D—Door, close it

3. Obtain portable audio equipment and samba or mambo music.

4. Create and practice a fire dance using the words in the four-step code and the rhythm of a samba or mambo beat. Use the rhythm to emphasize PPD _____ [facility's emergency number] and demonstrate the final *D* with a dip or swing of the hips.

Implementation

1. Distribute the Fire Dance Windowpane sheet to each participant.

2. Discuss the four emergency actions illustrated in the Fire Dance Windowpane, and identify the facility's emergency number.

3. Start the music and demonstrate your fire dance.

4. If you have a brave and fun group, ask them to join in the demonstration.

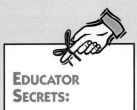

EDUCATOR
SECRETS:
This is great fun and
teaches important
content. Be prepared to
hear laughter.

By: Hal Vizino

FIRE DANCE WINDOWPANE

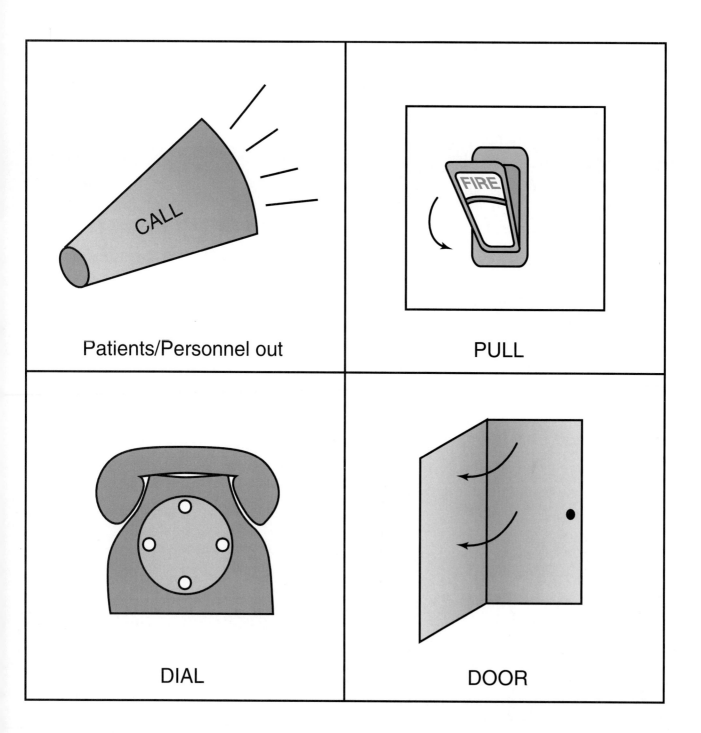

Patients/Personnel out

PULL

DIAL

DOOR

SAFETY SPIN TO WIN

TOOL BOX

Spin to Win Wheel,
Safety Spin to Win
Questions, Safety Spin
to Win Answer Key,
colored index cards,
colored markers,
scissors, paste or tape,
small prizes or goodies

Preparation

1. Copy the Safety Spin to Win Wheel and follow the directions to create the spinning wheel.

2. Identify desired colors to code content areas. For example, fire safety, pink; infection control, yellow; general safety, green.

3. Obtain markers and index cards in the selected colors.

4. Cut out Safety Spin to Win Questions and paste each question to the appropriate content color index card.

5. Separate the index cards into decks according to color.

6. Use markers to color code the wheel segments to correspond to the index card content color.

7. Assign a point value to each color.

8. Display the wheel where it can be easily seen by all participants (wall, flip chart, easel).

9. Collect small prizes or goodies (such as donuts, tootsie rolls, fruit snacks, pretzels, Post-it™ notes, etc.) to award to the participants at the end of the activity.

Implementation

1. Divide the group into two or more teams of three to six participants.

2. Assign each team a number.

3. Select a scorekeeper for each team.

4. Place color coded card decks on a table face down with each deck containing one color of cards.

continued

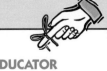

EDUCATOR SECRETS:

With only point values
on the wheel, it can be
used for a variety of
activities.

By: Elaine Hinojosa, MN, RNC

SAFETY SPIN TO WIN *continued*

5. Explain the following rules:

   a. Play starts with team one.

   b. The facilitator spins the Safety Spin to Win Wheel.

   c. When the arrow stops, the facilitator announces the color and point value for that wheel segment.

   d. The facilitator picks a card from the Spin to Win index cards that correspond to the color segment on the Safety Spin to Win Wheel where the arrow stopped.

   e. The facilitator reads the question.

   f. The team has 10 seconds to discuss the answer.

   g. A team spokesperson announces the answer. If the answer is correct, the team receives the points indicated on the Safety Spin to Win Wheel.

   h. If the answer is incorrect, the facilitator gives the other team(s) a chance to answer, or simply reveals the correct answers.

6. Use the Safety Spin to Win Answer Key to verify correct answers.

7. Total the team scores and award small prizes when play is completed or time has expired.

Note: Make sure all topic areas are covered at some time during the game.

8. Award prizes to all participants. Their knowledge has increased— They are all winners.

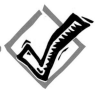

SAFETY SPIN TO WIN

Wheel

Directions:

1. Cut out the wheel and paste it to a piece of cardboard.

2. Do the same for the arrow.

3. Place the arrow on the wheel with a pivot paper clip.

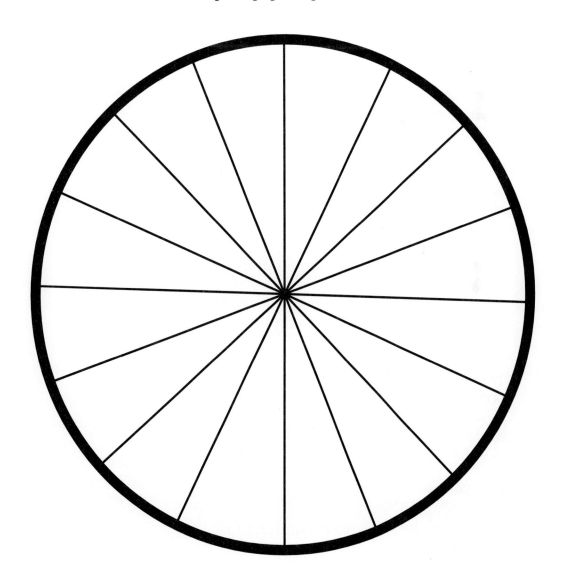

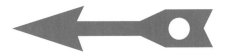

79

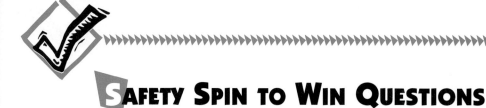

SAFETY SPIN TO WIN QUESTIONS

Infection Control and Bloodborne Pathogens

What are the two most significant bloodborne diseases to which you as a healthcare worker could be exposed to on the job, and by which are you more likely to be infected?

Name at least five ways you can safely perform your job and prevent exposure to bloodborne pathogens.

True or false: Make sure to store your food and drink close to you when working with blood so you don't have to leave the room.

What is the most widely used form of personal protective equipment in guarding against bloodborne pathogens?

What is one very basic way to prevent the spread of TB germs? (Hint: Your mama probably taught you this.)

Where should you be able to find the exposure control plan?

The fact that you may not be able to tell which patients carry a bloodborne pathogen requires you as a healthcare professional to do what?

Fire Safety

What does the *RACE* acronym stand for?

How do you report a fire?

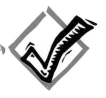

Safety Spin to Win Questions

General Safety, Including Electrical and Safe Medical Devices

What should you do for a person who is experiencing an electrical shock?

What does OSHA require on every label of a secondary container?

Name at least two actions that should prevent a patient with external cardiac pacing leads from experiencing a microshock, which is potentially fatal and may not even be felt by the patient.

What are the MSDS (Material Safety Date Sheets)?

Where are the MSDS located?

Is it a federal law or a hospital policy that requires us to report defective equipment on a Medical Device Report (MDR)?

What is an MDR reportable incident? What does this mean?

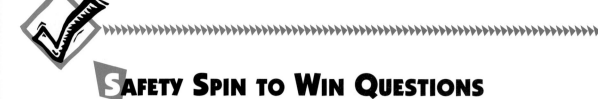

SAFETY SPIN TO WIN QUESTIONS

Answer Key

Infection Control and Bloodborne Pathogens

What are the two most significant bloodborne diseases to which you as a healthcare worker could be exposed to on the job, and by which are you more likely to be infected? *(Hepatitis B [HBV] and human immunodeficiency virus [HIV]; hepatitis B is the more likely infection.)*

Name at least five ways you can safely perform your job and prevent exposure to bloodborne pathogens. *(Safe handling of sharps. Proper use of sharps disposal. Proper handwashing. Do not bend, break, recap used needles. Proper handling of specimens. Cover cuts, rashes, etc. with gloves. No eating, drinking, lip balm where there are risks.)*

True or false: Make sure to store your food and drink close to you when working with blood so you don't have to leave the room. *(False; no food or drink should be stored where risk of contamination exists.)*

What is the most widely used form of personal protective equipment in guarding against bloodborne pathogens? *(Gloves. Wash hands upon removal, never wash or decontaminate single-use gloves, and remove glasses carefully so that no substance from soiled gloves contact your hands.)*

What is one very basic way to prevent the spread of TB germs? (Hint: Your mama probably taught you this.) *(Cover your mouth when you cough.)*

Where should you be able to find the exposure control plan? *(Infection control manual.)*

The fact that you may not be able to tell which patients carry a bloodborne pathogen requires you as a health care professional to do what? *(Use standard precautions and transmission-based isolation procedures; that is, treat all human blood and certain body fluids as if they were known to be infected with HIV, HBV, or other pathogens.)*

Fire Safety

What does the *RACE* acronym stand for? **(Rescue** the patient, **Alarm** activated, **Confine** the fire, **Extinguish** the blaze)

How do you report a fire? *(Pull the manual pull station and call the emergency operator.)*

continued

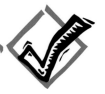

SAFETY SPIN TO WIN QUESTIONS

General Safety, Including Electrical and Safe Medical Devices

What should you do for a person who is experiencing an electrical shock? *(The victim may not be able to let go. Call for help. Check for responsiveness, initiate CPR, unplug and turn off the device.)*

What does OSHA require on every label of a secondary container? *(Chemical identification and appropriate hazard warning.)*

Name at least two actions that should prevent a patient with external cardiac pacing leads from experiencing a microshock, which is potentially fatal and may not even be felt by the patient. *(Avoid touching metal ends of leads, avoid touching other equipment, especially metal, and insulate leads with dry dressing, if not in use.)*

What are the MSDS (Material Safety Date Sheets)? *(Information from the manufacturer on the chemical hazards and how to control them, including: chemical and common names, ingredients, physical characteristics of chemical (odor, appearance, solubility in water), fire and explosion information, first aid, and symptoms of an overdose.)*

Where are the MSDS located? *(The employee right-to-know book.)*

Is it a federal law or a hospital policy that requires us to report defective equipment on a Medical Device Report (MDR)? *(Federal law, passed in 1991; the goal is to make manufacturers more accountable for the products they provide.)*

What is an MDR reportable incident? What does this mean? *(An MDR reports that a device contributed to the serious injury, death, or serious illness of a patient. For example: pumps, monitors, dressings, syringes, beds, IV lines [anything that is not a med], even operator error [because might help to detect a need for a change in design].)*

20-60 minutes

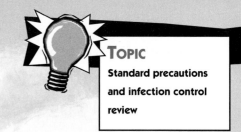
TOOL BOX

8½ × 11″ paper or large index cards, service bell, buzzer, flip chart or white board, marker, small prizes or goodies

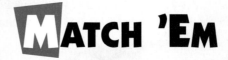

MATCH 'EM

Preparation

1. Identify mandatory topics to be reviewed. (Fire safety, infection control, etc.)

2. Write each topic (large print) on an 8½ × 11″ sheet of paper or large index card.

3. Compose questions to correspond to each selected mandatory topic.

4. Write each question on an 8½ × 11″ sheet of paper or large index card.

5. Obtain a service bell and a buzzer.

6. Set up a flip chart with easel and marker, or make sure you have access to a white board and marker. Use these for scorekeeping.

7. Collect small prizes or goodies (such as donuts, tootsie rolls, fruit snacks, pretzels, Post-it™ notes, etc.) to award to the participants at the end of the activity.

Implementation

1. Mix up the topic and question papers or cards.

2. Select an area (table or floor) where all can see, and place the topic and question papers or cards face down.

3. Arrange the papers or cards in rows with the same number in each row, forming a square when completed.

4. Select one participant to be your assistant, who should record points on the flip chart or white board, ring the bell for correct matches, and sound the buzzer for incorrect attempts.

5. Divide the group into two or more teams of three to six participants.

6. Invite the teams to select team names.

continued

EDUCATOR SECRETS:

Create a fun atmosphere. Encourage the selecting participant's team members to assist in the choosing process to minimize stress.

By: Teresa Colgan, BSN, RN, ET

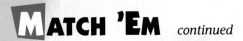

MATCH 'EM *continued*

7. Give the following instructions:

   a. The object is to match a question with the correct mandatory topic.

   b. Any team member from the team elected to go first picks and turns over two papers or cards to attempt a match.

   c. If a match is made you'll hear this sound—signal the assistant to ring the bell and the scorekeeper will record a point for the team.

   d. Play stays with the scoring team and card selection rotates among team members.

   e. If no match is made you'll hear this sound—signal the assistant to sound the buzzer—and play moves to the other team.

8. Continue play until all matches are made or until a designated time expires. The team with the highest score wins.

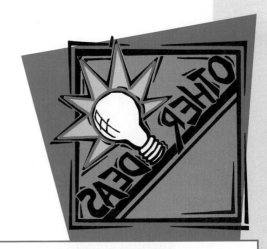

PART 3

INSTANT TOOLS FOR LEARNING IDEAS

20-30 minutes

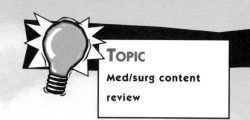
TOOL BOX

Two decks of playing cards with different-colored backing (such as one red and one blue), a list of content questions and answers

LET'S PLAY CARDS

Preparation

1. Select content for review that can be paired.

2. Type, cut, and tape to the face of the cards in deck number one questions on diseases, drugs, and physical findings. Place question content in the center of the card so the card's suit and value are visible.

3. Type, cut, and tape to the face of the cards in deck number two answers to correspond with deck number one. Place answer content in the center of the card so the card's suit and value are visible.

4. Examples of matches:

Deck #1	King of Hearts	Osteomyelitis
Deck #2	King of Hearts	Complication of open fracture
Deck #1	Queen of Hearts	Coumadin
Deck #2	Queen of Hearts	Oral anticoagulant
Deck #1	Jack of Hearts	Bucks traction
Deck #2	Jack of Hearts	Stabilizes hip fracture
Deck #1	Ten of Hearts	Red and yellow
Deck #2	Ten of Hearts	Two types of bone marrow
Deck #1	Nine of Hearts	PCA
Deck #2	Nine of Hearts	Method of pain control
Deck #1	Eight of Hearts	PTT
Deck #2	Eight of Hearts	Used to evaluate heparin therapy

continued

EDUCATOR SECRETS:

This provides a good review for content and concepts before testing. These decks can be reused.

By: Sandra H. Clark, RN, MSN

Let's Play Cards *continued*

Implementation

1. Present or review content.

2. Divide participants into groups or teams.

3. Shuffle the two decks together and distribute the cards equally.

4. Invite an individual or team to read a question card from deck #1. The individual or group with the answer responds.

5. Collect the matched pairs.

Variation

Ask the participants to shake hands on each match and return cards to the facilitator.

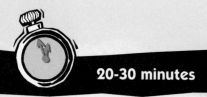

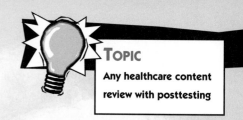

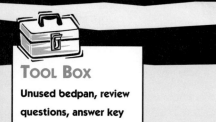

TOOL BOX

Unused bedpan, review questions, answer key

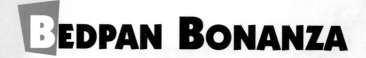

BEDPAN BONANZA

Preparation

1. Select content for review.

2. Make up questions to review major points, and prepare the appropriate answer key.

3. Type and cut out questions so that each question is on a single piece of paper, or print each question on an index card.

4. Place prepared questions in a bedpan.

Implementation

1. Teach desired content and remind participants that there may be a posttest.

2. Announce, "Yes, there is a posttest" when the teaching session is completed.

3. Walk around the room with the bedpan containing the questions held high.

4. Allow each participant to reach into the bedpan and pick out a question.

5. Allow 3 to 5 minutes for participants to research the answer.

6. Have all participants, one at a time, read their questions and answers to the group.

7. Remind participants to listen and take notes.

Variation

Divide participants into teams for competition.

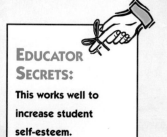

EDUCATOR SECRETS:

This works well to increase student self-esteem.

By: Nancy Moulaison, RN, BSN

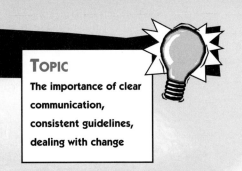
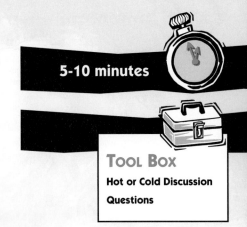

TOOL BOX
Hot or Cold Discussion Questions

HOT OR COLD

Preparation

1. Copy the Hot or Cold Discussion Questions.
2. Select the debriefing questions that will make the learning point you desire.

Implementation

1. Recruit a volunteer who is willing to do this activity in front of a group of people.
2. Separate the volunteer from the group by having him or her step out in the hall.
3. The group selects three activities for the volunteer to do or objects for the volunteer to find.
4. Invite the volunteer back into the room.
5. Explain the rules. Round 1: If the volunteer comes close to doing the activity or finding the object, the group responds, "hot." If the volunteer is not doing the activity or moving away from the object, the group responds, "cold."
6. Ask the volunteer to begin.
7. Round 2: Direct the group to respond only with "hot" when the volunteer becomes close to the object or activity.
8. Round 3: Direct the group to respond only with "cold" when the volunteer moves away from the object or activity.
9. The volunteer usually becomes frustrated and no longer wants to participate.
10. Discuss with the group the major learning points about the activity.

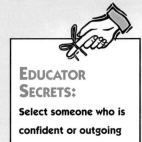

EDUCATOR SECRETS:
Select someone who is confident or outgoing as the volunteer.

By: Linda Chitwood, RN, MS

HOT OR COLD

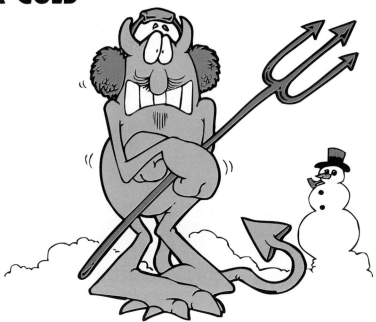

Discussion Questions

Select some of the questions listed below to debrief this activity and to make the desired learning point. You can adapt this list or make up your own questions.

1. How long did it take the volunteer to respond correctly in Round 1?

2. How did the volunteer respond in Round 1, hearing both hot and cold clues?

3. How did the volunteer feel in Rounds 2 and 3?

4. How did the observers feel in Rounds 2 and 3?

5. Did the volunteer quit at any point in the activity? Why?

6. How important is it to communicate clearly and simply?

7. Was the volunteer able to reach the goal easily in Rounds 2 and 3? Why or why not?

8. How do Rounds 2 and 3 relate to change in an organization?

9. Have you ever experienced a situation in your job similar to this activity? What happened?

10. How important is clear communication?

11. How important is it to give consistent guidelines and instructions?

12. Does this activity simulate what it feels like when in the midst of change?

13. What are some of the tools we can use to deal effectively with change?

14. How does this activity relate to your job or your life?

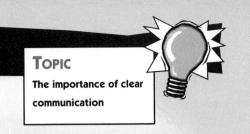

5-10 minutes

MIXED MESSAGES

TOOL BOX
Mixed Messages?
Figures 1 and 2, Mixed
Messages? Questions
for Discussion,
overhead projector or
flip chart with easel
or white board, paper,
pens or pencils

Preparation

1. Copy Mixed Messages Figures 1 and 2. If using an overhead projector, make transparencies. If using a flip chart, copy one figure to a page. If using a white board, do not draw the figures until the activity begins, and make sure the board can easily be seen.

2. Select the debriefing questions that will make the desired learning points.

Implementation

1. Divide participants into pairs.

2. Identify one participant of each pair as *A* and the other as *B*.

3. Request A's and B's to stand back to back. Participants A faces the front of the room, participants B faces the back of the room.

4. Distribute paper and pencil to participants B, and instruct them NOT to turn around.

5. Display Mixed Messages? Figure 1.

6. State that participants A will have 90 seconds to describe a figure to participants B, and participants B must draw the figure without asking questions. Participants B must remain silent.

7. Call time when 90 seconds is up, and have participants B compare their drawings to the displayed one.

8. Ask for a show of hands for how many pictures matched exactly.

9. Have the pairs trade places. A's face the back of the room and B's face the front.

10. Distribute paper and pencil to participants A.

11. Display Mixed Messages? Figure 2.

continued

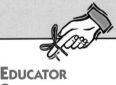

EDUCATOR SECRETS:
Select a participant who is confident or outgoing to describe the figure first.

By: Michele Deck, RN, MED, BSN, ACCE-R

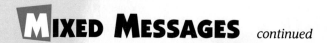

MIXED MESSAGES *continued*

12. State that participants B will have 90 seconds to describe the next figure to participants A, and participants A must draw the figure without asking any questions. Participants A must remain silent.

13. Call time when 90 seconds is up, and have participants A compare their drawings to the displayed one.

14. Ask for a show of hands for how many pictures matched exactly. You should see a slightly higher percentage.

15. Discuss with the group the major learning points about the activity by selecting questions from Mixed Messages? Questions for Discussion.

Variation

Select one participant to describe the figures to the group and have each member of the group draw the figures.

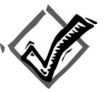

MIXED MESSAGES?

Figure 1

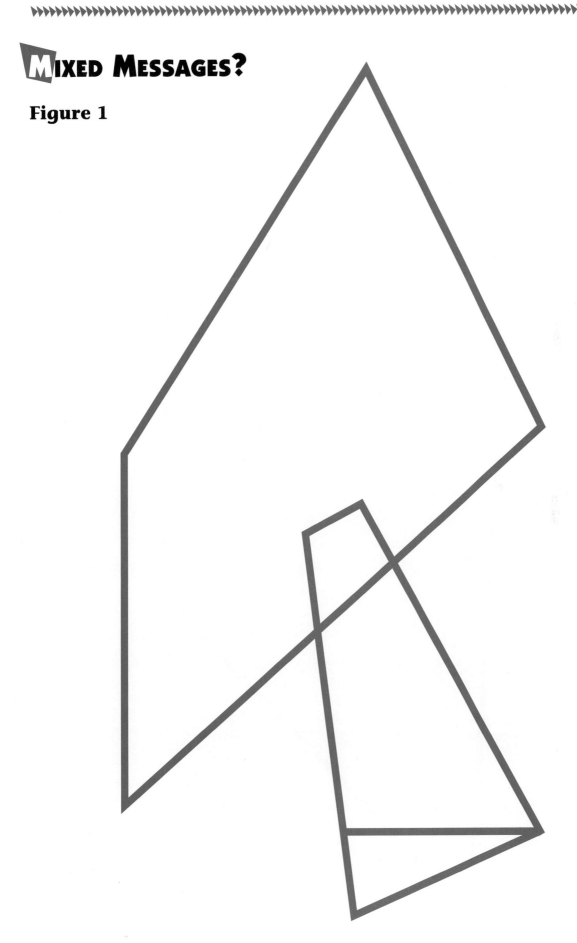

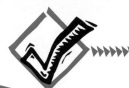

MIXED MESSAGES?

Figure 2

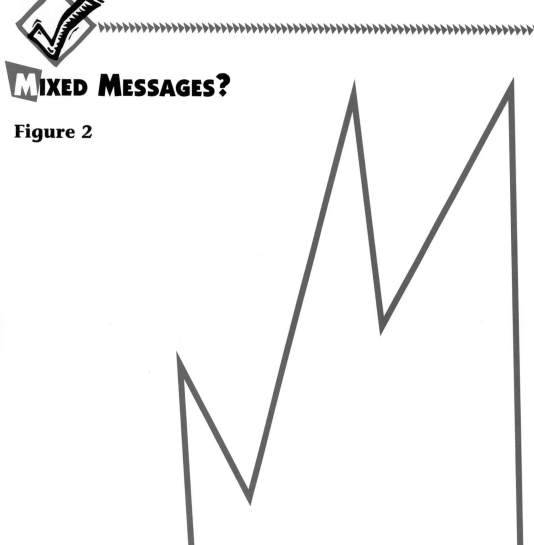

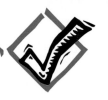

MIXED MESSAGES?

Questions for Discussion

1. How did it feel to be the person drawing?

2. How did it feel to be the person describing the figure?

3. Did you feel you were a better "drawer" or "describer"? Why?

4. Is it possible to misunderstand directions? Why?

5. What were the barriers to effective communication?

6. What factors enhanced communication in this activity?

7. This activity demonstrates one-way communication. In your job or life, what are some of the circumstances in which you give one-way communication?

8. What are some of the circumstances in which you receive one-way communication?

9. Is it possible that others misunderstand directions? Why?

10. If you were to repeat this activity, what new rules would you add to enhance the chance of all reaching success?

11. How does this activity relate to your life or your job?

12. What are five learning points this activity illustrates about effective communication?

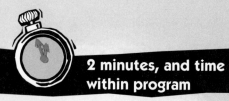

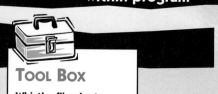

TOOL BOX

Whistle, flip chart, marker, police hat and badge, pens or pencils

TOPIC

Any healthcare content where unfamiliar terms or acronyms are used, including computer training, physical assessment, quality improvement, JCAHO, etc.

JARGON POLICE

Preparation

1. Determine your group size. You may need to assign additional Jargon Police representatives for groups of 40 or more participants.

2. Obtain one police hat and badge for each Jargon Police representative.

3. Set up flip chart with marker.

4. Obtain whistle.

Implementation

1. Explain that it is essential for everyone to be familiar with the vocabulary associated with the selected healthcare content.

2. Appoint or recruit one volunteer per group (40 or less participants) to act as the Jargon Police representative.

3. Hand out a badge, hat, and whistle to each Jargon Police representative, and state "You are now deputized."

4. Instruct participants to notify the Jargon Police whenever an unfamiliar word or term is encountered. Notification can be by a raised hand or a handwritten note passed to the Jargon Police.

5. Instruct the Jargon Police to blow the whistle when notified and call for clarification.

6. Define the identified word or words, and have the Jargon Police keep a running list of terms and meanings on the flip chart. Recording terms and meanings helps participants remember what has been "policed" and provides a reference that can be hand copied and used for review.

7. Make a note of any words you have difficulty defining, and, if possible, research the answer over break and announce the answer to participants when the session resumes.

Variation

Jargon Police can wait until several words have been accumulated to blow the whistle and call for clarification.

EDUCATOR SECRETS:

Distribute a list of words that are frequently encountered as a glossary the next time you teach the same content.

By: Pamela Brown Stewart, MN, RN, CCRN

BALLS AROUND THE CIRCLE

TOOL BOX
Three different small,
soft balls per large
group (Nerf, Koosh);
Balls Around the Circle
Debriefing Questions

Preparation

1. Determine your group size. If your group is larger than 40 you may need to break the group into two teams with three balls each.

2. Copy the Balls Around the Circle Debriefing Questions.

Implementation

1. Invite participants to stand in a close circle.

2. Give directions for Round 1: Instruct the participants to throw the ball to one other. Each person must catch and throw the ball only once.

3. Ask participants to remember who threw them the ball.

4. Ask participants to remember to whom they threw the ball.

5. Make sure everyone understands the directions.

6. Start Round 1 by throwing one of the balls as described above.

7. When the last participant receives the ball, it returns to the facilitator.

8. Round 2: Instruct the group members to throw the ball in the same pattern, only faster.

9. Round 3: Repeat the pattern, even faster!

10. Round 4: Start a second ball in the circle after the first ball has begun. Then add a third ball.

11. Be prepared to see chaos, confusion, and dropped balls.

12. Debrief the group using the Balls Around the Circle Debriefing Questions.

EDUCATOR SECRETS:
A fifth round can be done with a focus on making sure participants can catch the ball when it is thrown.

By: Pamela Brown Stewart, MN, RN, CCRN

BALLS AROUND THE CIRCLE

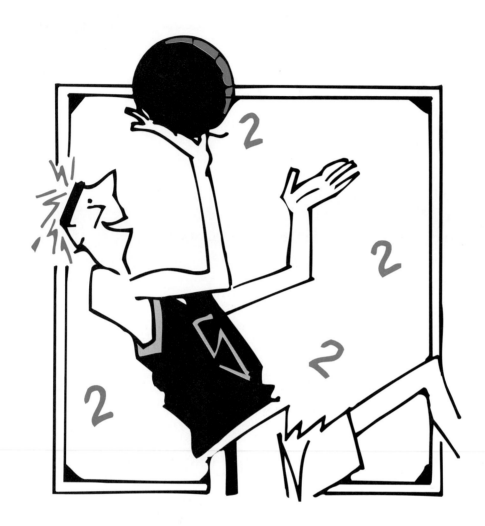

Debriefing Questions

1. What caused the simple task of passing the balls to become more difficult or complex?

2. What happened to the stress level as multiple variables were added to the situation?

3. How did stress impact performance?

4. How did you feel as the stress increased?

5. What learning lesson can we take from this activity?

6. How does this relate to our jobs and our lives?

7. If we were to do this task again, what could we do to decrease the stress level?

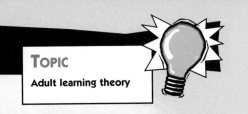

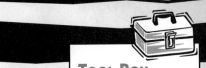

BRINGING ADULT LEARNING THEORY TO LIFE

TOOL BOX

Post-it™ notes or paper, flip chart with easel, colored markers, masking tape

Preparation

1. Gather necessary tools.
2. Be aware of the six fundamental principles of adult learning according to adult learning theory:
   a. Need to know
   b. Readiness to learn
   c. Orientation to learning
   d. Self-concept
   e. Learner's experience
   f. Motivation to learn

Implementation

1. Have each participant identify two reasons for choosing to attend your class or seminar.
2. Invite participants to form groups of four or five, and combine reasons.
3. Write or recruit a scribe to write on the flip chart using large print.
4. Record one or two reasons from each group, or until you have enough reasons to provide examples of the six principles of adult learning.
5. Tape the flip chart pages to the walls or doors, whatever space is available, where they are visible to all participants.
6. Explain a principle of adult learning, then have participants choose examples from the flip chart pages that reflect that concept.
7. Give other examples to connect principles of adult learning to the classroom and life-long learning.

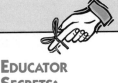

EDUCATOR SECRETS:

Make sure you have enough flip chart pages up for all groups to discuss, one per team.

By: Mary Beth Swaboda, MSN, RN, CCRN

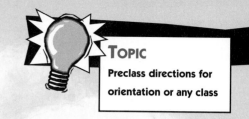

TOOL BOX

Colored 8½″ × 11″ paper; tape; large, flat men's shoe

FOLLOW THE FOOTPRINT

Preparation

1. Gather supplies listed in the Tool Box.
2. Place large, flat shoe on a sheet of 8½″ × 11″ paper.
3. Trace the outline of the shoe. This is your pattern.
4. Copy the foot pattern on colorful paper. The number needed depends on the distance to the location to which you are leading.
5. Use the same footprint pattern for right and left prints. The footprint turned to one side provides a right footprint, and turned to the other side a left footprint.

Implementation

1. Tape footprints from the door or elevator to the class directory board.
2. Tape more footprints from the board to the classroom.

Variation

You can record positive messages on the footprints, such as:

Good morning!

Walk this way.

Follow me!

Welcome to our class.

We are so glad you came to class today!

EDUCATOR SECRETS:

This combats confusion when classes change classrooms, and acts as an energizer.

By: Mary Beth Swaboda, MSN, RN, CCRN

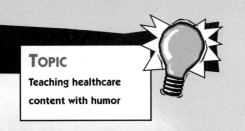

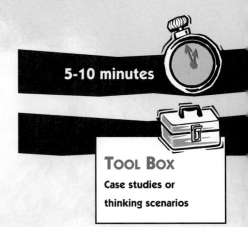

TOOL BOX

Case studies or
thinking scenarios

"IN CASE"D IN FUN

Preparation

1. Select a case study or thinking scenario.
2. Replace the names with some of the names listed below:

   Warren Peace, MD

   Dee Argee

   Sam Tort

   Constance Care

   Marion Haste (marriage counselor)

   Cheatem N. Howe

   Willy B. Good

   Cy Bernet

   F. Stop Fitzgerald

   Denton Fender

   Chester Drawers

   Bjorn Touloose

   Clara Phyll

   Cathi Puroheart

   M.T. Jarr

Implementation

1. Present the case studies or thinking scenarios as planned.
2. Discuss key content points.

EDUCATOR
SECRETS:

This works well to add a
little humor to some
serious content points.

By: Mary Arnone Cahoon, BS, RN

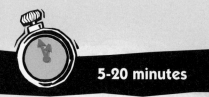

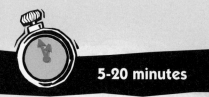

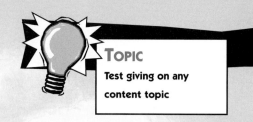

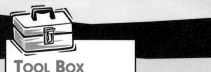

TOOL BOX
Test questions, small adhesive labels, miniature chocolate candy bars, container to hold candy bars

TASTY TESTS

Preparation

1. Compose questions that apply to the content of the planned learning session or program.

2. Type test questions onto adhesive labels. (Suggest: $1'' \times 2\frac{5}{8}''$ adhesive labels.)

3. Obtain miniature chocolate candy bars, at least one for each participant.

4. Attach one question to each miniature candy bar.

5. Place all the "question bars" into a container.

Hint: Keep a small supply of diabetic chocolates.

Implementation

1. Present the planned content.

2. Ask each participant to draw a "question bar" from the container.

3. Have everyone, one at a time, read his or her question aloud and state the answer. If the answer is incorrect, encourage others in the group to help their classmate provide the correct answer.

4. Instruct the participant who gives the correct answer to collect their classmate's "question bar," and keep it as his or her prize. (Similar to the game "Rob your Neighbor.")

Variation

Divide the group into small teams and have the team spokesperson announce the answers.

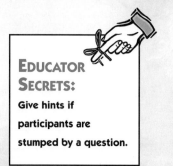

EDUCATOR SECRETS:
Give hints if participants are stumped by a question.

By: Mary Arnone Cahoon, BS, RN

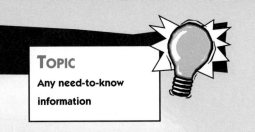

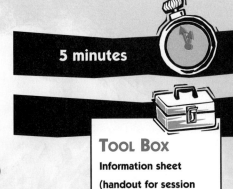

5 minutes

TOOL BOX
Information sheet
(handout for session
content)

HAVE TO **K**NOW **I**NFO

Preparation

1. Develop a one-page "information sheet" handout. The information sheet should include key information participants need to know to be successful in their work environment. The information sheet should focus only on the "need-to-know" content.

2. Provide references on the handout so participants can read more about the information noted.

3. Copy one information sheet for each participant.

Implementation

1. Distribute the information sheet to each participant.

2. Explain major points covered on the information sheet.

3. Invite the participants to take the information sheet home and suggest they use it as an on-the-job reference.

EDUCATOR SECRETS:
Request assistance from others on your management team to determine where the greatest needs are, for example, what types of info the staff "forgets."

By: Mary Arnone Cahoon, BS, RN

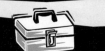

TOPIC
Leadership approaches, essential components: communication, trust, understanding, commitment, shared vision

COLLABORATION PUZZLE

TOOL BOX

Jigsaw puzzles of 60 to 80 pieces (one per team); picture of completed puzzle; Collaboration Puzzle Faciliator Reference sheet; Collaboration Directions 1, 2, and 3; envelopes for each puzzle (optional)

Preparation

1. Determine your group size.

2. Provide one 60 to 80 piece jigsaw puzzle and a picture of each completed puzzle per team of four to six participants. Puzzles can be left in their original boxes or placed in envelopes for easy traveling. Whatever method you choose, it is important to include a picture of the completed puzzle.

3. Review and copy the Collaboration Puzzle Faciliator Reference sheet, and select which Collaboration Directions sheet or sheets you will need.

4. Make copies of the Collaboration Directions sheet or sheets for each team member.

Implementation

1. Divide your group into small teams of four to six participants.

2. Select a team leader for each team, and invite the leaders to come to the front of the room.

3. Take the team leaders out of the room or form a tight circle or huddle so they can receive directions without the other participants hearing what is said.

4. Distribute puzzle boxes or envelopes to the team leaders and explain the following: "Everything you need to complete the assigned task is included in the box/envelope. Directions are included. Give each of your team members a copy of the directions." When the task is complete, you will be asked to summarize how your group responded to the assignment.

5. Have the team leaders return to their teams.

continued

EDUCATOR SECRETS:

Relax and enjoy whatever happens. You can tie actions and reactions to learning points.

By: Pamela Brown Stewart, MN, RN, CCRN

COLLABORATIVE PUZZLE *continued*

6. Give the following direction to the entire group: "Your team leader is returning with a task for each team to complete. Begin when you receive the directions. I will tell you when to stop."

7. Signal the group to stop work when one team completes their task.

8. Ask each team leader to stand and read their directions and describe how their team approached the task, team member attitudes, and comments. If you have a large group, limit the team leader debrief to each Collaboration Directions and puzzle setup combination listed on the Collaboration Puzzle Faciliator Reference sheet.

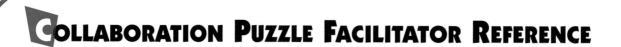

COLLABORATION PUZZLE FACILITATOR REFERENCE

Use as many collaboration directions and puzzle setup combinations as you wish, depending on the number of teams.

Collaboration Directions 1: Productive

Puzzle Setup	Level of difficulty
Correct puzzle picture	Easy
Incorrect puzzle picture	Difficult
No puzzle picture	Very difficult

Collaboration Directions 2: Less productive

Puzzle Setup	Level of difficulty
Correct puzzle picture	Moderately difficult
Incorrect puzzle picture	Difficult
No puzzle picture	Very difficult

Collaboration Directions 3: Least productive

Puzzle Setup	Level of difficulty
Correct puzzle picture	Difficult
Incorrect puzzle picture	Very difficult
No puzzle picture	Extremely difficult

Comments

Each group will approach this exercise in their own way. Do not try to influence the process or outcome. If a team decides to do nothing, you may suggest they take a break or start to fill out the program evaluation. However, they should not interfere with the work of another team.

When the team leaders describe what happened on their team, you may find that particular colors or edge pieces were assigned to specific individuals. You might say, "Oh, you formed a task force."

COLLABORATION PUZZLE FACILITATOR REFERENCE

Build desired learning points from this activity. For example, some teams, especially those with Collaboration Directions 2—very difficult and Collaboration Directions 3—any level of difficulty, may choose to do nothing. In the debrief or summary you can discuss how this response is common, especially when a large task is communicated through a memo with very little instruction or support. Those teams where only one person can talk should have lots to say, too.

Expand on any trends toward competitiveness or anger that the teams demonstrate.

An interesting event sometimes occurs when it is time to break up the puzzles and return them to their box or envelope. Some groups have trouble doing this. You may comment, "It's hard to break up something we put our energies into" or "Coming up with new ideas and ways to do things is often easier than letting go of old ideas/ways."

For discussion, begin by stating, "Being a star in your organization through effective collaboration involves five components that are demonstrated by the puzzle activity. Use these discussion points to reinforce collaboration:

- **Shared vision:** Everyone understands the task/outcome. Without shared vision, people may see things differently. Shared vision is represented by the puzzle picture included with the puzzle activity.

- **Understanding roles and responsibilities:** People contribute differently in collaboration. We can't "keep score" (i.e., all contribute the same). This component is represented by the collaboration directions received with each puzzle activity identifying the roles of group members.

- **Communication:** Collaboration mandates skilled communicators. This is represented by the collaboration directions.

- **Trust:** People working together must trust one another in a variety of ways (confidentiality, respect for opposing ideas, etc.). The collaboration directions either facilitate or work against trust.

- **Commitment:** This component is evidenced in the collaboration directions by "quitting" and collaboration directions given to support the group's ability to complete the task. Some are committed and have poor directions/vision, yet they have great outcomes.

109

COLLABORATION DIRECTIONS 1

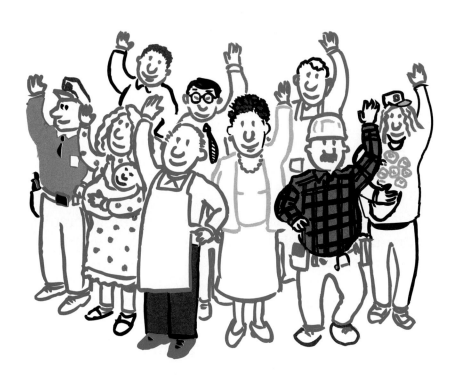

1. The group's task is to work together to assemble this easy puzzle.

2. A picture of the puzzle is provided, so you will all have a vision of what it is you will be creating.

3. You were assigned to this group because of your skill and ability to work with others.

4. You may use whatever method or technique you desire to accomplish your task.

5. All members of the group should be comfortable with their contribution. Do your best.

6. You may use whatever resources you have or can obtain to accomplish this task.

7. You may begin when everyone in the group has these directions. Good luck!

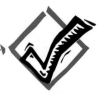

COLLABORATION DIRECTIONS 2

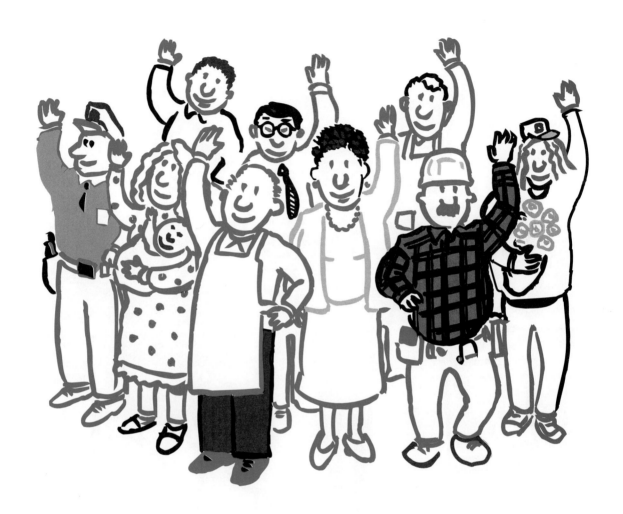

1. Your group's task is to assemble the puzzle pieces given here.

2. Only one person in your group may speak to the group leader in accomplishing this task.

3. Your group is not expected to accomplish very much.

4. You may quit whenever you like.

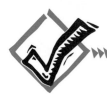
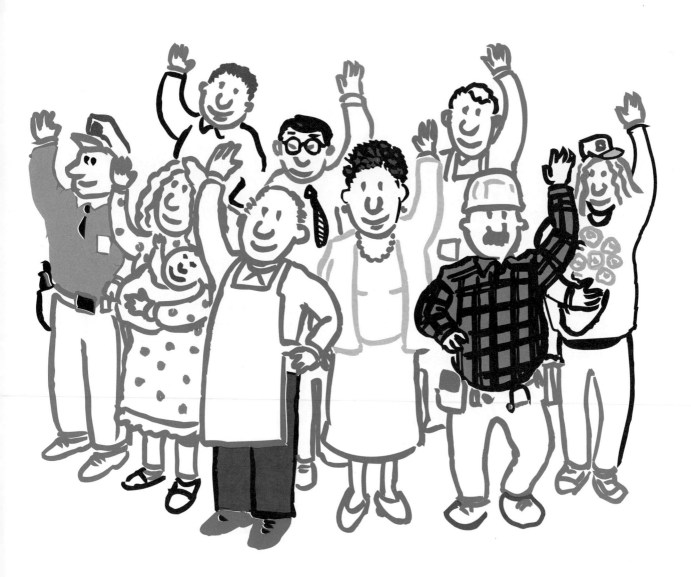

Go for it!

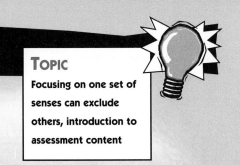

TOPIC

Focusing on one set of
senses can exclude
others, introduction to
assessment content

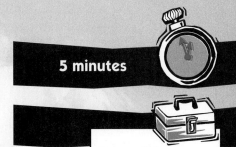

5 minutes

TOOL BOX

Duo Intros Questions,
watch with second hand
or timing device, paper,
pencils or pens

DUO INTROS

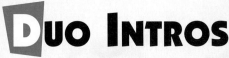

Preparation

1. Select the desired discussion questions from the Duo Intros questions.

2. Have on hand a watch with a second hand or timing device.

3. Make sure all participants have paper and pencil or pen.

Implementation

1. Divide your class into duos (twosomes).

2. Ask duos to select who will be *A* and who will be *B*.

3. Invite participants A to begin by talking for 90 seconds about the best vacation they ever had.

4. Ask B to take in as much as possible about A.

5. Call time after 90 seconds.

6. Ask participants B to share for 90 seconds their favorite vacation.

7. Ask A and B duos to stand back to back.

8. Distribute paper and pencil to each participant.

9. Ask each participant to make a list of 10 physical characteristics about his or her partner. They can't look, and the description must be as specific as possible, such as blue eyes, white blouse, etc.; not vague, such as nice smile.

10. Give the learners one to two minutes to make their lists.

11. Say, "I know you want to list 20 things, but please stop now!" (There may be some laughter.)

12. Ask participants to share their lists with their partners.

13. Ask how many duos had a completely accurate list.

14. Discuss the learning points you have selected from the Duo Intros Questions.

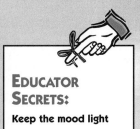

EDUCATOR
SECRETS:

Keep the mood light
and fun.

By: Michele L. Deck, RN, MEd,
BSN, ACCE-R

113

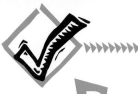

Duo Intros Questions

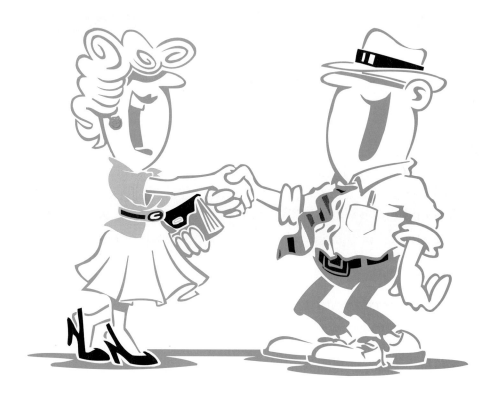

1. How many duos had 10 accurate physical characteristics?

2. Were you surprised when asked to make a list of physical characteristics? Why?

3. How many of you were focused so hard on listening that you didn't pay attention to the appearance of your partner?

4. Have any of you seen a similar activity in which you must listen carefully and then introduce your partner to the class?

5. Does previous experience or expectations affect the results of this activity?

6. How does this activity relate to your job?

7. What important points does this remind us of involving physical assessments and our need to use all our senses equally?

8. What are some of the secrets or shortcuts you use when doing a physical assessment?

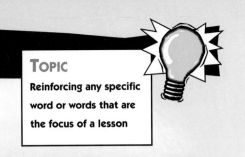
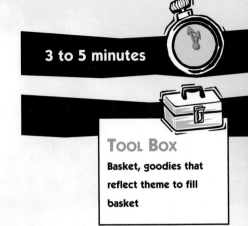
WORD BASKET

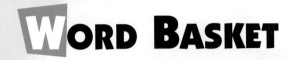

Preparation

1. Obtain a small basket.

2. Fill the basket with a selection of goodies that reflect the topic or lesson. Some possibilities include: Fire balls or red hots for fire safety, smarties for test reviews, soaps for infection controls, foil-covered chocolate coins for budget presentations, Lifesavers for CPR.

3. Select your key word or words.

Implementation

1. Display the basket in the front of the room before you begin the lecture or presentation.

2. Pick up the basket and place it on a participant's chair (select at random).

3. Explain the following directions: "The person who has the basket is invited to listen along with everyone else for the 'key' word or phase, which is _____. When the person in possession of the basket hears the key word or phrase, she or he must select one thing from the basket and pass the basket on to someone else in the class."

4. Begin your lecture or presentation. The passing continues throughout the room until your presentation is over. This encourages everyone to pay attention. If the temporary basketholder misses a saying of the key word or phrase, the classmates will remind him or her.

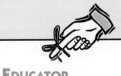

By: Michele L. Deck, RN, MEd, BSN, ACCE-R

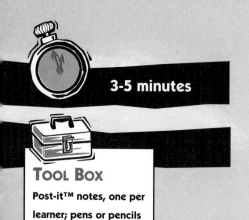

3-5 minutes

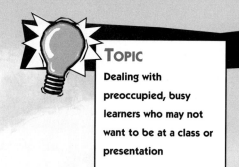

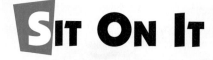

SIT ON IT

Preparation

1. Obtain Post-it™ notes, one per person.
2. Obtain pens or pencils.

Implementation

1. Invite each person to obtain a Post-it™ note before you begin the lecture or presentation.
2. Begin by asking the participants to write down on the Post-it™ note something currently on their minds that could get in the way of their learning.
3. Ask the participants to stand when they are finished writing, with the Post-it™ note in hand.
4. Invite the participants to reach under their chairs and attach the Post-it™ note to the underside of the chair.
5. Ask everyone to sit down.
6. Suggest to the participants that for just a short time they will have to "sit on" these thoughts or concerns. This active demonstration allows the mind to let go or put aside distractions for a short period of time.
7. Invite participants to take their Post-it™ notes with them at the end of the class or presentation.

EDUCATOR SECRETS:

Acknowledging competing elements in attention allows participants to know you appreciate their demanding lives.

By: Michele L. Deck, RN, MEd, BSN, ACCE-R

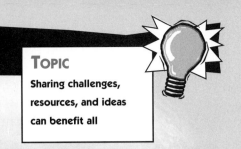
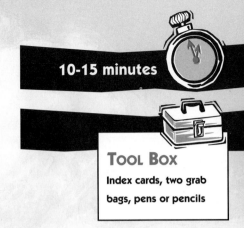

QUESTION AND ANSWER BAG

Preparation

1. Obtain two index cards for each participant.

2. Obtain two grab bags. Label one "Questions" and the other "Answers."

3. Have extra pens or pencils available for those who do not bring one.

Implementation

1. Option: Divide your group into small teams, if you are using a team approach.

2. Distribute two index cards to each participant or team scribe.

3. Begin by asking the participants or team scribes to write down on one index card a question or challenge they face.

4. Collect these in the Questions bag.

5. Invite the participants or team scribes to write down on the other index card a possible answer or solution to the question or challenge they previously recorded.

6. Collect these in the Answers bag.

7. Ask each participant or scribe to reach in the Questions bag and Answers bag and select one index card from each.

continued

EDUCATOR SECRETS:
You may be amazed at the accuracy of randomly selected answers.

By: Michele L. Deck, RN, MEd, BSN, ACCE-R

QUESTION AND ANSWER BAG *continued*

8. Ask each participant or team scribe to read his or her selected question first and the selected answer second. One of two results will occur. The answer may indeed fit the question and be appropriate. This will surprise everyone. The other outcome is the answer to the question will be so mismatched it will be funny.

9. Continue until all have shared their selected questions and answers, or intersperse the question and answer reading at intervals throughout the presentation.

10. Make the point that sometimes others have the answers to our questions or solutions to our mutual challenges.

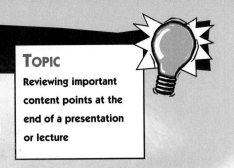

TOPIC
Reviewing important
content points at the
end of a presentation
or lecture

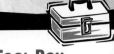

5-15 minutes

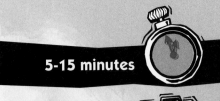

TOOL BOX
Four to six sheets of
flip chart paper,
masking tape or
adhesive, water-based
markers, four to six flip
chart easels (optional)

MEMORY CHARTS

Preparation

1. Test the paper with the markers to make sure they do not bleed through.

2. Hang blank sheets of flip chart paper at four to six locations around the meeting room or classroom, using masking tape or adhesive of some kind. As an option, use four to six flip chart easels with pads located throughout the room.

3. Make sure that you have at least one marker per participant.

Implementation

1. Present your content or lecture.

2. Distribute one marker to each participant at the completion of your information.

3. Ask the participants to visit each of the flip chart sheets or easels, writing in marker one key point they learned from the presentation.

4. Instruct participants not to duplicate learned points. Each entry must be a new idea.

5. Have each participant visit each flip chart page at least twice.

6. Begin the activity by saying, "Ready, Set, Go!"; participants will find themselves racing to and from charts, writing at the same time as others.

7. Review the items as they are recorded. If any key learning points do not appear, you can reintegrate this information.

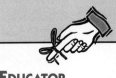

EDUCATOR SECRETS:
The participants will not only review the information, but will naturally compete to have fun.

By: Michele L. Deck, RN, MEd, BSN, ACCE-R

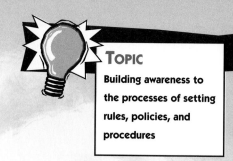

TOOL BOX

Rules and Policies for Construction sheet, building blocks (different colors, shapes, and sizes), bags or boxes to hold blocks, timing device, pens or pencils

RULES AND POLICY CONSTRUCTION

Preparation

1. Determine the number of participants, and divide into teams of three to seven participants.

2. Obtain building blocks in different sizes, shapes, and colors. You need a set of building blocks for each team and each set should contain 20 to 30 blocks.

3. Place each set of building blocks in a bag or box.

4. Copy one Rules and Policies for Construction sheet for each team.

Implementation

1. Divide the group into small teams of three to seven participants.

2. Distribute a bag of building blocks to each team.

3. Have each team select a scribe to record on the Rules and Policies for Construction sheet.

4. Distribute Rules and Policies for Construction sheet to each team scribe.

5. Explain the following:

   a. Each team will write four policies or rules for building a structure using the blocks.

   b. Provide some examples, such as, "Builders can only use one hand to hook pieces together," or "No two blocks of the same color can be connected."

   c. The team scribe is to write the rules or policies on the Rules and Policies for Construction sheet.

   d. When each team has completed writing the rules and policies for the construction project, the written rules and policies will be passed to another team, and that team will need to build their project following the written rules and policies.

continued

EDUCATOR SECRETS:

This activity creates awareness of the importance of input in setting rules and policies.

By: Pam Brown-Stewart, MN, RN, CCRN

RULES AND POLICY CONSTRUCTION *continued*

6. Allow the teams two to four minutes to come up with the construction rules.

7. Have the teams exchange rules.

8. Begin the activity by saying, "Ready, Set, Go!"

9. Give the teams five minutes to work on their construction project.

10. Stop the activity and discuss the difficulties in trying to follow rules and policies you had no part in creating.

11. Ask the group to discuss parallels between this exercise and challenges they face on the job.

Variation

At step 7 in the process, announce to the group that you made a mistake, and each team will use their own rules and policies. Ask the team if they knew the rules would be theirs to follow, would the rules be different? Why does this happen? Can they relate this exercise to a job or life challenge?

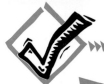

RULES AND POLICIES FOR CONSTRUCTION

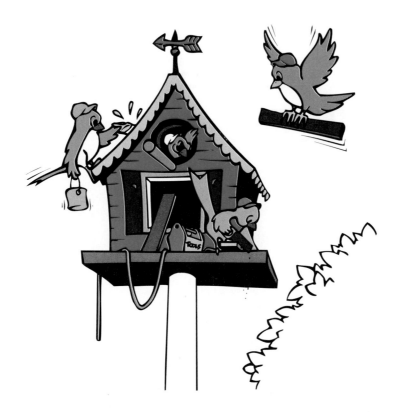

1. All team members must be involved in the placement of the pieces.

2. Everyone must begin together when the educator says, "Go!"

3. The team must have a goal of what the construction will be at completion.

4. At least 20 building blocks must be used.

Create four additional rules/policies:

1. _____

2. _____

3. _____

4. _____

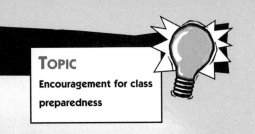
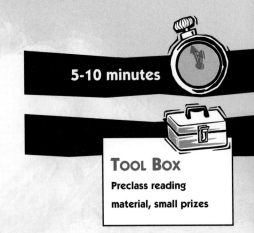

TOOL BOX

Preclass reading material, small prizes

READING BETWEEN THE CLUES

Preparation

1. Ready preclass reading material to include a secret word located within the content.

2. Follow these steps:

   a. On the cover of your materials attach a colorful Post-it™ note that says, "If you are willing to read this material before class, you will find a hidden prize inside."

   b. On page two in the middle of a paragraph include the following sentence, "You've found the first clue, keep reading!"

   c. Halfway through the reading material place another sentence that says, "You are almost there; keep reading!"

   d. About three-quarters of the way through the material, place another sentence that says, "Congratulations! You have found the secret word! When you come to class, tell me the secret word *football* and you will receive a special prize. Don't share the secret word with anyone but me."

3. Obtain prizes desired by participants. (Hint: Facility vendors are sometimes willing to contribute free promotional items.)

Implementation

1. Distribute preclass reading material to participants three to four days before the class meets.

2. Make sure you arrive at class a bit early so that you are available to participants.

3. Award a prize to the first participant that notifies you that the secret word is *football*.

4. Watch for the other participants' reaction to the prize. Comments may be heard regarding the prize source. Hopefully, the award recipient will comment on the preclass assignment.

5. Remember: Change the secret word and its location for each new class assignment.

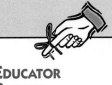

EDUCATOR SECRETS:

The word will pass quickly that there is a good reason to arrive at class prepared.

By: Michele L. Deck, RN, MEd, BSN, ACCE-R

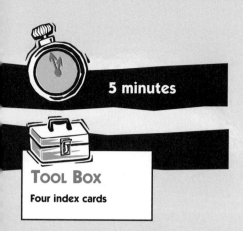

TOOL BOX

Four index cards

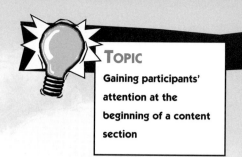

TOPIC

Gaining participants' attention at the beginning of a content section

PARTICIPANT ANNOUNCERS

Preparation

1. Obtain four index cards.

2. Label each card as 1, 2, 3, and 4.

3. Print or type the words, "Good morning," or "Good afternoon," whichever applies to your class or presentation time, on index card 1.

4. Print or type the words, "Welcome to _____ class" on index card 2.

5. Print or type a sentence that describes what the class or presentation is about, such as, "Today we will learn a four-step process to deal with a fire emergency" on index card 3.

6. Print or type the words, "Turn to page one in the handout and let's begin" on index card 4.

7. Hand out the index cards randomly to four participants as they enter the room.

Implementation

1. Explain the following to your group: "Four people received index cards when they arrived at class. Those four people face a decision. They can stand if they are willing to read the card, or they can hand the card off to someone else who is willing to read the card."

2. Ask those willing to read to stand up.

3. Ask the person who has card #1 to read the card aloud. When finished, have the reader request the participant holding card #2 to read his or her card aloud. This continues until all 4 cards are read. When the 4 cards have been read, the participants have provided the introduction to the content.

Hint: You can also put your personal introduction material on the card instead of content.

EDUCATOR SECRETS:

Allow the participants to choose to read or hand off. Not everyone is a natural talker or reader.

By: Michele L. Deck, RN, MEd, BSN, ACCE-R

TOPIC
Encouraging all people at different levels and jobs throughout your facility to put those divisions aside so that they can work effectively together

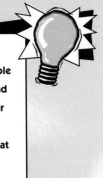

5-10 minutes

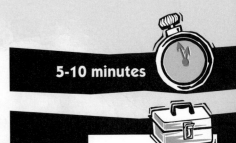

TOOL BOX
Index cards, decorated gift bag with handle, pens/pencils

CHECK YOUR TITLES AT THE DOOR

Preparation

1. Obtain a least one index card per participant.

2. Purchase or make a nicely decorated bag.

3. Have extra pens or pencils available.

Implementation

1. Distribute index cards to learners at the beginning of your class or presentation.

2. Ask everyone to write down their current title or job position title on the index card.

3. Collect the index cards in the gift bag.

4. Explain that for today, you are taking the titles and placing them outside the door of the classroom or meeting room.

5. Walk over to the door, open it, and place the bag just outside the door.

6. Emphasize that for the educational session's time frame, our new title is "Learner." This helps to show that all learners are of equal importance today, removing set mind barriers to different levels working together effectively.

Reminder: At the end of the class or presentation, all can reclaim their titles as they leave the room, if desired.

EDUCATOR SECRETS:
This increases learner comfort and ability to work effectively together.

By: Michele L. Deck, RN, MEd, BSN, ACCE-R

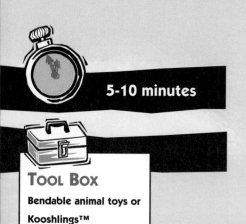

TOPIC
Encourage participants
to become aware of
their feelings about
change, challenges, and
acknowledging these
feelings

ANIMAL ANTICS

Preparation

1. Obtain at least one bendable animal toy or Kooshling™ per participant or team.

Implementation

1. Divide your group into teams, if you are using a team approach.

2. Distribute bendable animal or Kooshling™ to each participant or small team at the beginning of your class or presentation.

3. Ask the participants or teams to reflect on how they feel about change in the organization at this moment.

4. Invite the participants or teams to pose the animal or Kooshling™ to reflect this identified feeling.

5. Ask them to show the pose and tell the entire group or small team about what the animal reflects.

6. Present your content on change, the quality process, or dealing with challenges in the organization.

7. When your class or presentation is half over, ask them to repose the animal or Kooshling™ if their feelings have changed since the beginning.

8. At the end of the class or presentation, ask for a repose of the animal or Kooshling™ if their feelings have changed since the last description.

9. Wrap up discussion points with positive changes in feelings of those who have expressed them.

EDUCATOR SECRETS:

Model this activity by using and showing your animal or Kooshling™ to show you empathize with the participants.

By: Michele L. Deck, RN, MEd, BSN, ACCE-R

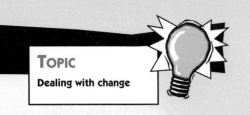
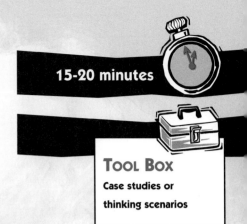

CHANGE CARPET

Preparation

1. Create a "paper carpet" from white butcher paper with room enough for your group members to stand. (Thirty feet long is a good length for 15 to 20 people.)

2. Label segments laid end to end: Denial, Resistance, Adaptation/Exploration, and Commitment.

3. Prepare content on the change process in relation to the four stages of change (Denial, Resistance, Adaptation/Exploration, and Commitment).

Implementation

1. Introduce the four stages of change, describing and discussing each.

2. After the discussion, ask the participants to stand on the paper carpet space that best describes where they are in the change process.

3. Ask the following questions and foster a discussion:

   Why did you choose this stage?

   Will your choice likely change from day to day?

   How can we help each other move toward commitment?

   Does it help to know where others are in the change process?

4. Wrap up discussion points with positive changes strategies expressed by members of the group.

EDUCATOR SECRETS:

Be cautious, this creates awareness and deals with feelings that can be powerful.

By: Hal Vizino

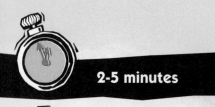
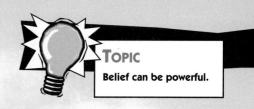
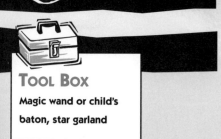

TOOL BOX

Magic wand or child's baton, star garland

MAGIC WAND

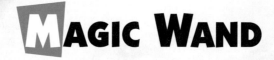

Preparation

1. Buy a magic wand or create one from a child's baton. (If you use the child's baton, pull off one end of the baton's streamers and attach a star burst made from star garland.)

Implementation

1. Use the wand for various purposes. For example, ask, "Who makes the magic?" during a program. Or touch people with it and say, "There—You now possess the magic to accomplish your task!"

2. Use this gimmick for programs on stress, time management, and change. It's great!

EDUCATOR SECRETS:

Watch how people relate this prop to important learning points.

By: Hal Vizino

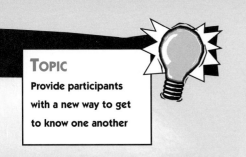

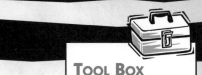

Sweet Introductions

Preparation

1. Buy snack packs of M&Ms, one per person or one small pack per team.

2. Make a poster or overhead transparency of the following discussion points.

Brown: Favorite food

Green: Something you want to learn during this program

Yellow: Something of which you are afraid

Red: Something that embarrasses you

Orange: Favorite hobby

Blue: Something of which you are proud

Variation: Use the colors to review important information, such as:

Brown: One important learning point from the session

Green: One idea you've learned that you will use back on the job

Yellow: What you learned that surprised you

Red: One barrier that will make it difficult to implement your new knowledge

Orange: Your favorite class quote or event

Blue: One thing about which you'd like to learn more

Implementation

1. Divide your group into teams of two to six participants.

2. Provide each team with a small bag of M&Ms or one snack pack per person. If you have one small pack for a group, ask someone to begin by opening the bag and dumping out a few for themselves, and then pass the bag so that everyone can do the same.

continued

EDUCATOR SECRETS:

For those who don't like sweets, stress they must tell the fact but can give away the candy.

By: Hal Vizino

Sweet Introductions *continued*

3. Ask the participants to refrain from eating the M&Ms until they are told to do so.

4. When all have selected their candies, inform the participants that for each M&M selected, they are to share certain information about themselves or the content.

5. Display the prepared overhead.

6. Invite each participant to begin by stating his or her name and then giving the information that corresponds to the color of the M&Ms held.

7. Allow participants to eat the candy after they share the requested information.

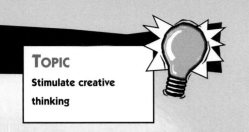

TOPIC
Stimulate creative
thinking

5-10 minutes

OLD SHOE STIMULATION

TOOL BOX
Any object that can
stimulate thought, such
as an old shoe, a
newspaper, an apple, a
sponge, a chocolate
bar, or screwdriver

Preparation

1. Select and obtain the object to be presented to participants.
2. Identify the problem the participants will work on.

Implementation

1. Explain to participants that a totally unrelated piece of information can help bring restructuring to an established pattern. Both concepts and the problem are held in attention. Connections eventually form between the two diverse concepts.

2. Stimulate discussion by saying, for example, "How is this shoe like our challenge?" Offer a first connection such as, "The problem has a sole."

Note: This can be conducted as an open class session with participants making suggestions as to how the object may be related to the problem, or it can be discussed in groups.

EDUCATOR SECRETS:
Give small teams
different objects and
the same challenge, and
see interesting results.

By: Hal Vizino

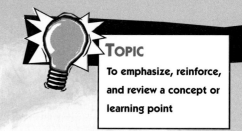

TOOL BOX

Sound device, such as a ratchet, cowbell, tunemaker, or train whistle

PAVLOV'S NIGHTMARE

Preparation

1. Select and obtain the sound device to be presented to participants.
2. Identify the concept to be emphasized or reinforced that corresponds to the sound.

Implementation

1. Introduce a concept word or action, and use the sound device to make the corresponding sound effects. For example, for an EKG course, when saying the concept "monitor rhythm," sound a rap ball that makes rhythmic sounds. Or, in a customer service program, every time a phone ringing sounds, everyone must smile.
2. Connections eventually form between the sound and the concepts or action.

Suggestion: Use more than one sound or action for each concept.

EDUCATOR SECRETS:

Use a maximum of four or five sounds in a program. Sounds will add fun and energy to any session.

By: Hal Vizino

132

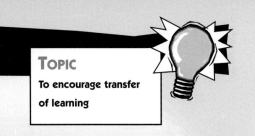
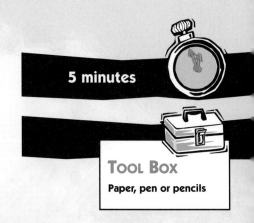
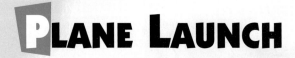

PLANE LAUNCH

Preparation

1. Obtain paper and pen or pencils.

Implementation

1. Distribute one piece of paper to each participant.

2. Make sure each participant has a pen or pencil.

3. Invite participants to write their name, title, address, and telephone number on the paper.

4. Ask them to write down one thing they learned that they plan to implement as soon as possible, and a date when they plan to implement it.

5. Ask each participant to make his or her paper into an airplane.

6. Gather the group into a large circle and have them launch their airplanes simultaneously toward the circle's center.

7. When the planes land, ask each person to retrieve one paper airplane and sit down.

8. Invite the participants to read the information on the paper plane selected, noting the name, date, and idea to be implemented.

9. Ask each person to call his or her "plane person" one week after the date listed, and discuss how implementation of the skill or knowledge proceeded.

EDUCATOR SECRETS:

This creates responsibility and bonds between peers to actually use something they have learned.

By: Hal Vizino

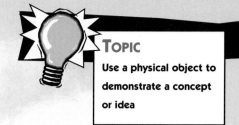

TOOL BOX

A slippery tube (it looks like a brightly colored hot dog that has puckered ends and is water filled)

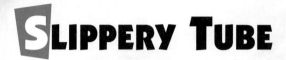

SLIPPERY TUBE

Preparation

1. Obtain slippery tube toy.

Implementation

1. Ask participants to stand, and inform them that they will have something to catch and to throw to each other.

2. Throw a slippery tube to a participant, and request that she or he throw it to another participant. Many participants will not be able to hold onto the tube, and it will slip out of their hands. It may feel strange, cold, or clammy to some.

3. Stop the action after several throws and ask, "What does this tube represent?"

4. Offer this point: Sometimes a skill or subject area is hard to grasp and hold on to. That's why we're here today: to learn how to get a hold on the *subject!*

EDUCATOR SECRETS:

Observe participants' reaction to the object, and reflect those points when discussing the exercise.

By: Hal Vizino

TOPIC

Information relating to the pharmacy department and administration of medication protocols for staff nurses in a new facility

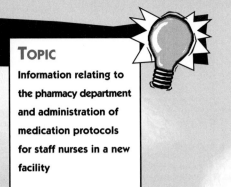

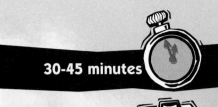

TOOL BOX

Rebus Puzzle, backboard or corkboard (approximately 32" × 40"), 24 cards (thin cardboard cut to approximately 6" × 7½"), velcro

MEDICATION MATCHES

Preparation

1. Copy the Medication Matches Rebus Puzzle, or create one of your own. You can use a poster copy machine to increase the size.

2. Tape or use push pins to attach the rebus puzzle to a backboard or corkboard.

3. Select 12 medication items and their corresponding descriptor. (For example, NAR: narcotic administration record.)

4. Cut thin cardboard to make 24 cards, approximately 6" × 7½" each.

5. Write the 12 medication items on the cards, one medication item to each card.

6. Write the 12 corresponding descripters on the remaining cards, one descriptor to each card.

7. Scramble the two card sets (medications and descriptors) together randomly.

8. Number the blank side of the cards, leaving cards in random sequence, from 1 to 24. (IMPORTANT: Be sure to apply numbers **after** the cards have been scrambled.)

9. Place a small piece of velcro on the top side of the medication/descriptor side of each card.

10. Place a small piece of velcro on your rebus puzzle board where the medication/descriptor cards will be attached to cover the puzzle picture clues.

11. Arrange the cards in numerical order on the puzzleboard. (Numbers to the outside, medications/descriptors face down.)

continued

EDUCATOR SECRETS:

Cards can be made on colored paper to assist participants in making matches. Remember to shuffle the colored paper before you write medications and descriptors.

By: Elaine Hinojosa, RN, MN

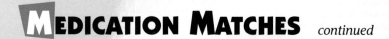

MEDICATION MATCHES *continued*

Implementation

1. Divide participants into two or more teams.

2. Elect or appoint a spokesperson for each team.

3. Select a team to go first.

4. Ask the team spokesperson to pick a number reflected on one of the cards (a number from 1 to 24).

5. Turn the card with the selected number over and read it to the group.

6. Ask the team to consult on the second number selection and have the team spokesperson announce the number.

7. Turn over the card with the selected number, and read it to the group. There are two possible results:

   a. **Match**—If the two cards turned over match (medication and descriptor), the cards are removed from the board and the choosing team has 10 seconds to guess the rebus puzzle statement.

   b. **No match**—If the cards turned over do not match, the cards are placed back on board in their original positions.

8. Move play to the next team with either outcome.

9. Explain the significance of both components (medication and descriptor) when a match is made.

10. Show and explain any matches not completed at the time the puzzled is solved.

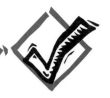

MEDICATION MATCHES

Rebus Puzzle

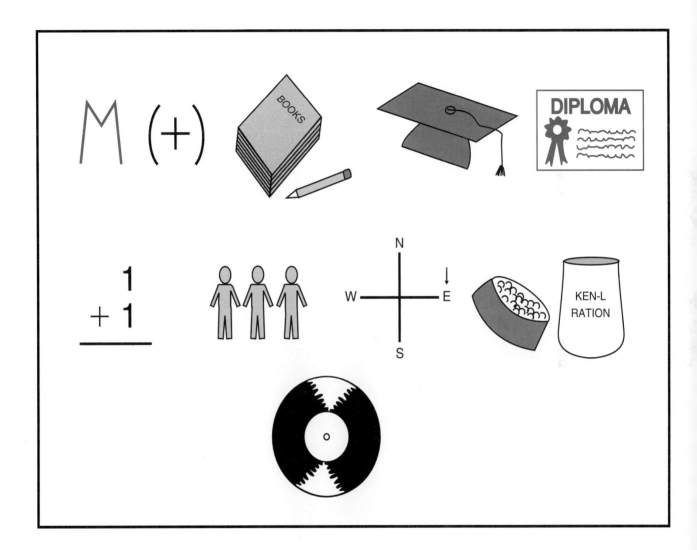

Rebus puzzle idea:
Medication administration record

M + Education

Add + men + east + ration

Record

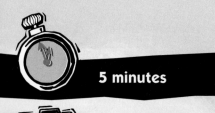

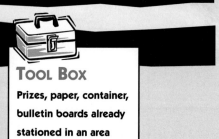

TOOL BOX

Prizes, paper, container, bulletin boards already stationed in an area

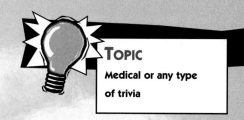

TOPIC

Medical or any type of trivia

BRAIN TEASING MEDICAL TRIVIA

Preparation

1. Label a container "trivia responses."

2. Establish an area on a bulletin board, and label it "brain teasing medical trivia."

3. Post guidelines on the bulletin board for participation:

   a. Submit answers into the "trivial response" container.

   b. The first correct answer [date entries] or the most correct answer receives a prize.

   c. Correct answers and prize winners will be posted.

   d. Post time element of each game.

   e. Have fun!

Implementation

1. Collect the answers daily.

2. Post the correct answers and winners at the end of the time frame.

3. Distribute prizes to winners.

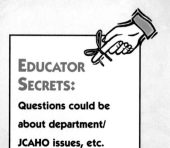

EDUCATOR SECRETS:

Questions could be about department/ JCAHO issues, etc.

By: Penny Gorman, BSN, RN

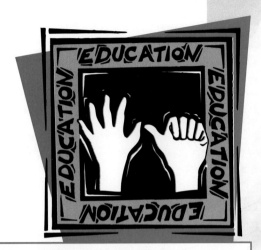

PART 4

INSTANT TOOLS FOR CURRICULUM AND CONTINUING EDUCATION

30 minutes

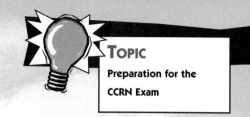
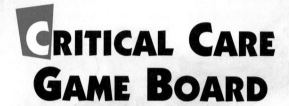

CRITICAL CARE GAME BOARD

TOOL BOX

Critical Care Game
Board; one die; CCRN
exam review book;
index cards and markers
in the following colors:
white, red, green,
yellow, purple, and blue

Preparation

1. Copy Critical Care Game Board.

2. Color the Critical Care Game Board squares alternating the
   following colors: white, red, green, yellow, purple, and blue.

3. Obtain a die from an old game or a game store.

4. Set up the Critical Care Game Board in an area where all can see.

5. Obtain a CCRN question and answer review book, select desired
   questions, and color code to correspond to the code categories
   listed in step 6.

6. Obtain and label colored index cards (these are your category
   cards) as follows:

   White—Neuro

   Red—Cardiovascular

   Green—Gastrointestinal

   Yellow—Renal

   Purple—Pulmonary

   Blue—Miscellaneous

Implementation

1. Divide participants into even teams.

2. Display the category cards where all can see the category and
   corresponding color.

3. Pick a team to go first by rolling a die (highest number goes first).

4. Ask each team to find an item from their pocket, purse, or
   organizer that can be used as a playing piece.

5. Place all playing pieces on START.

continued

**EDUCATOR
SECRETS:**

This can be used to
review any type of
content before an
exam.

By: Jana Magarelli, RN, MA

CRITICAL CARE GAME BOARD *continued*

6. Have a team representative roll the die and move the team playing piece the same number of squares as the number rolled on the die.

7. Note the color of the square where the playing piece lands, and select a question from the CCRN review book that corresponds to that category color.

8. Read the question. If the team answers correctly, their playing piece stays on the space where it landed. If the team answers incorrectly, the playing piece moves back to the space where it was before the die was rolled.

9. Play continues until one team or all reach the finish.

Optional: Prizes can be awarded to all participants. Their knowledge has increased; they are all winners.

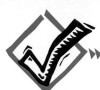

CRITICAL CARE GAME BOARD

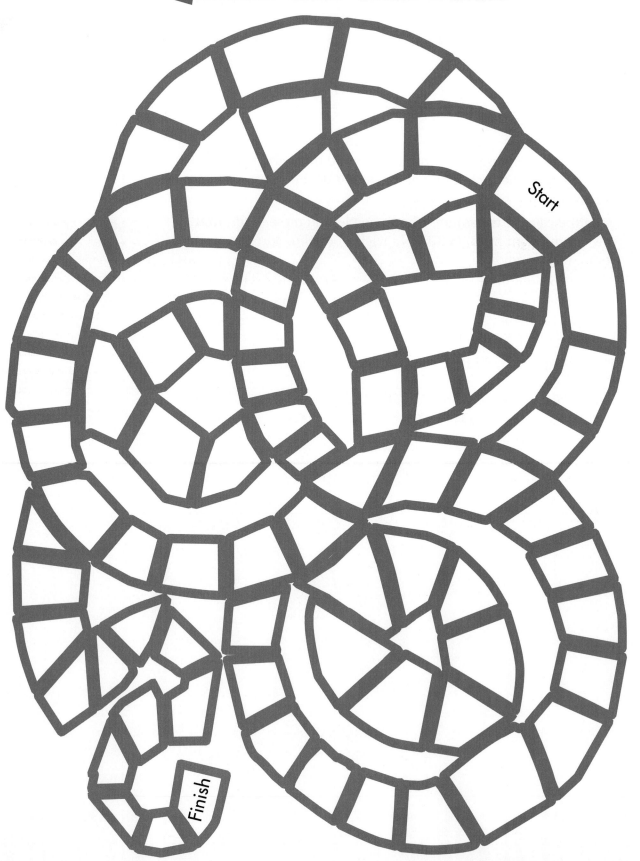

Start

Finish

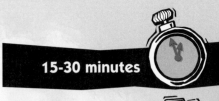

LURKING LATEX!

Preparation

1. Determine the number of participants and divide the group into teams of two to four participants.

2. Copy Lurking Latex Allergy Type and Reaction sheet for each team. Each sheet equals a set.

3. Cut each boxed item on the Latex Allergy Type and Reaction sheet into a single strip.

4. Place each cut set into an envelope, one envelope for each team.

5. Copy Lurking Latex Overhead Transparencies 1, 2, and 3 to overhead transparency sheets.

6. Place Post-it™ notes over each small square on Overhead Transparency 2.

7. Copy the Lurking Latex Bingo Cards, one for each participant. Use a variety of cards.

8. Collect for each team latex items or hypoallergenic latex items used in and around the participants' worksite, and place the items in paper bags. Provide one bag per team.

9. Design a Lurking Latex bouquet. Blow up balloons, condoms, gloves, etc.

10. Prepare a flip chart, and list methods of exposure, high risk groups, and types of reactions. Use Lurking Latex Allergy Type and Reaction sheet as a guide.

Implementation

1. Display the Lurking Latex bouquet.

2. Discuss the need for latex allergy education, and use Overhead Transparency 1 to stress this issue.

3. Divide participants into teams of two to four participants.

4. Distribute paper bags containing the Lurking Latex items to each team.

continued

By: Susan Duly, BSN, CNOR, RN
Penny Gorman, BSN, RN

LURKING LATEX! *continued*

5. Invite the teams to search the bags for any item that does not contain latex. (Remember: All items collected contain latex.) Stress that hypoallergenic doesn't mean free of latex.

6. Display the prepared flip chart list and discuss the methods of exposure and high risk groups. (Hint: Use storytelling to expound on this issue.)

7. Show Overhead Transparency 2, Lurking Latex Windowpane.

8. Uncover one windowpane square at a time while asking the group what they think each picture represents. (Hint: Occasionally, review those already revealed for reinforcement.) Use the answer key as a guide.

9. Show Overhead Transparency 3. Randomly select a square and ask participants to recall the symptom represented by that square. Use the answer key as a guide.

10. Distribute one envelope containing cut Lurking Latex Allergy Type and Reaction strips to each team.

11. Invite participants to work as a team to organize the Lurking Latex Allergy Type and Reaction strips; that is, match the allergic reaction with the corresponding symptom. This exercise provides a review of the information discussed and listed on the flip chart.

12. Reveal the correct answers.

13. Use a blank flip chart page to brainstorm on patient care and staff issues concerning latex allergies.

14. Distribute Lurking Latex Bingo Cards, one card for each participant.

15. Explain that the winner must yell, "Latex" when a complete line is marked horizontally, vertically, or diagonally.

16. Call the numbers L-5, A-20, T-34, E-44, and X-59, along with a few random numbers to make the appearance of a real game.

17. All should yell "Latex" at the same time.

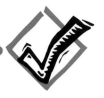

LURKING LATEX ALLERGY TYPE AND REACTION

Directions: Copy and cut apart on the lines. Place the strips in envelopes, one envelope for each team.

Irritant

Dryness and cracking

Aggravated by glove powder

Dryness

Nonallergic

Type I

Urticaria

Wheezing, respiratory difficulties

Systemic

Anaphylactic shock

Type IV

Never systemic

Puritis

Redness and cracking

Delayed reaction

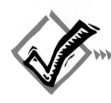

DELIVERY MAN OCCUPATIONAL HAZARD

Overhead Transparency 1

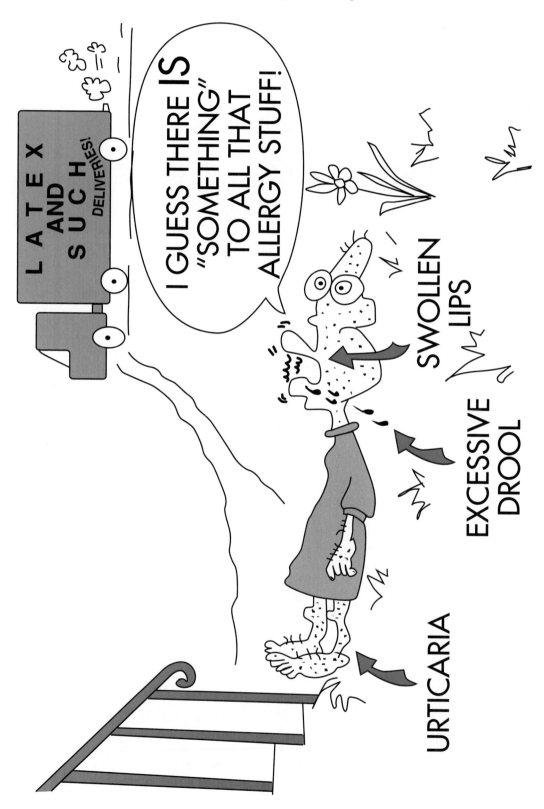

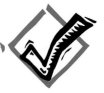

LURKING LATEX WINDOWPANE

Overhead Transparency 2

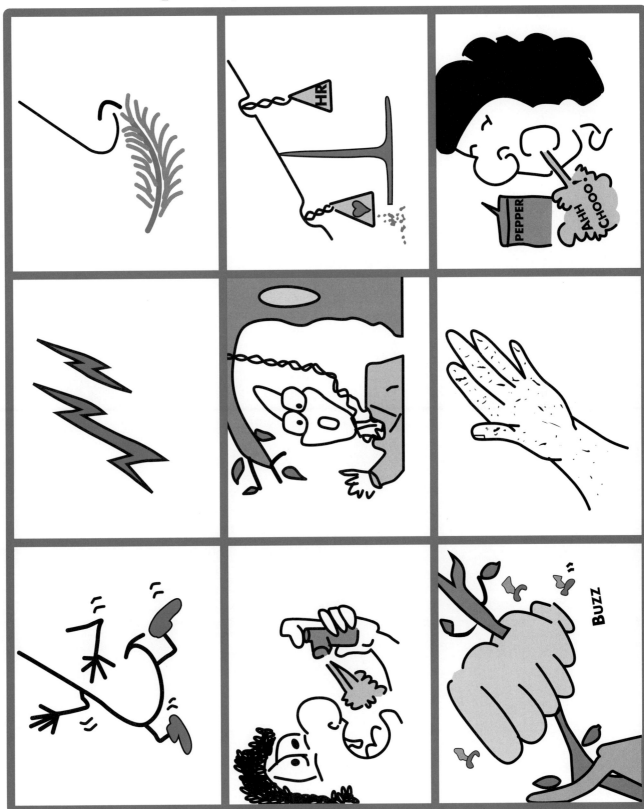

147

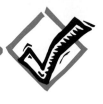

LURKING LATEX BLANK WINDOWPANE

Overhead Transparency 3

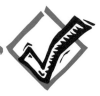

LURKING LATEX WINDOWPANE

Answer Key

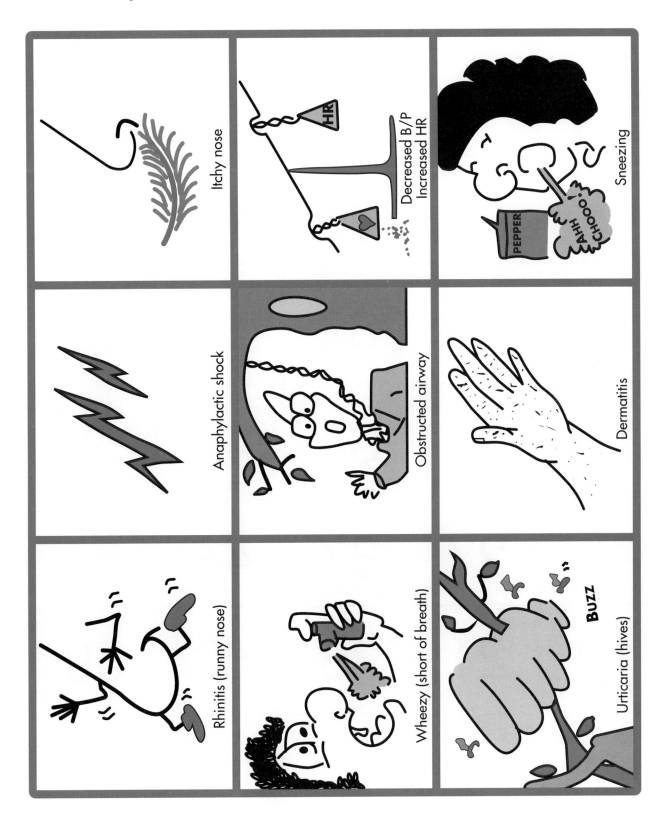

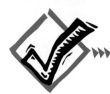

LURKING LATEX BINGO CARD

L	A	T	E	X
5	24	38	41	53
7	20	32	49	52
19	26	34	47	55
8	27	37	44	57
13	21	35	42	59

LURKING LATEX BINGO CARD

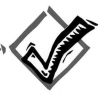

L	A	T	E	X
1	25	30	47	53
18	21	31	45	60
5	20	34	44	59
14	29	33	40	51
6	22	39	48	56

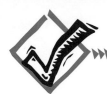

LURKING LATEX BINGO CARD

L	A	T	E	X
11	23	33	47	50
16	25	39	49	53
4	22	30	40	51
10	28	38	42	55
5	20	34	44	59

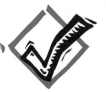

Lurking Latex Bingo Card

L	A	T	E	X
2	27	30	41	59
17	26	38	44	60
9	21	34	47	52
12	20	39	48	54
5	29	35	40	57

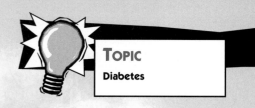

TOOL BOX

Syringes and saline, anatomical arm or oranges, blood glucose monitor, sample foods (real or synthetic), carbohydrate table, other nutrition materials, instruction cards

CAN YOU CUT IT AS A DIABETIC

Preparation

1. Prepare a lecture on the various aspects of diabetes:
   a. Meal planning and nutrition
   b. Insulin injections
   c. Blood glucose monitoring
   d. Activity
   e. Physical challenges
   f. Anatomy and physiology of diabetes

2. Create instruction cards, one per participant. The card should include:
   a. Type of diabetes
   b. Physical condition
   c. Type of medication prescribed
   d. Age, weight, and other similar information

3. On a side table, set up syringes and saline, anatomical arm or oranges, blood glucose monitor, sample foods (real or synthetic), carbohydrate table, and other nutrition materials.

Implementation

1. Participants are told they have diabetes and are given an instruction card.

2. Present the lectures or discussions as outlined above.

3. Participants must assume the role of the patient described on the card for the day.

4. After break, ask the participants what they ate on break and in what activities they engaged.

5. Challenge the participants to defend their food and activity choices as appropriate to their instruction card.

6. Ask the learners to plan the evening meal, and stick to it.

continued

EDUCATOR SECRETS:

Be in tune to the participants' ability to think like a diabetic patient.

By: Mary Ann Jones, MA, RN

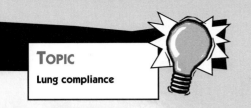
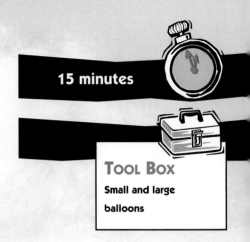
COMPLIANCE BALLOONATHON

Preparation

1. Obtain one small and one large balloon for each participant.

Implementation

1. Distribute one small and one large balloon per participant.

2. Ask participants to blow up the small balloon.

3. Ask them to note how much pressure in general terms it takes to get some air volume in the balloon. (Is it easy or hard?)

4. Now invite participants to blow up the larger balloon.

5. Ask them to estimate how much pressure it takes to blow up the larger balloon.

6. Discuss the issue of patient lung compliance. A patient with decreased lung compliance has lungs that are stiff and hard to inflate, like the small balloon. The larger balloon, which is easier to inflate, helps demonstrate how patients with increased lung compliance takes less pressure to get a certain volume of air into their lungs.

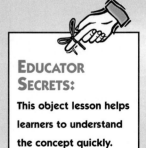

EDUCATOR SECRETS:

This object lesson helps learners to understand the concept quickly.

By: Mary LaBiche, MEd, RRT

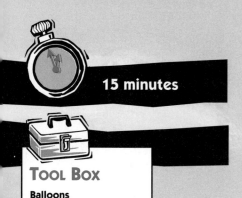

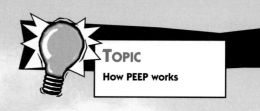

PEEP GOES THE BALLOON

Preparation

1. Obtain one balloon per participant.

Implementation

1. Distribute one balloon per participant.
2. Ask participants to blow up the balloon.
3. Have participants deflate the balloon, leaving a small amount of air in the balloon.
4. Invite participants to again blow up the balloon with the air already in it.
5. Use this to demonstrate how PEEP works in patients: An alveoli that is collapsed and contains no air is hard to inflate. This is why PEEP is used. It helps to keep the alveoli open (as the partially inflated balloon illustrates) and makes it easier for the patient to breathe.

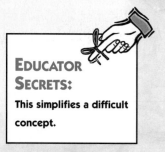

EDUCATOR SECRETS:

This simplifies a difficult concept.

By: Mary LaBiche, MEd, RRT

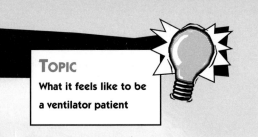

TOPIC
What it feels like to be
a ventilator patient

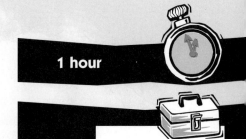
TOOL BOX
Ventilator, endotracheal
tubes (one per
volunteer)

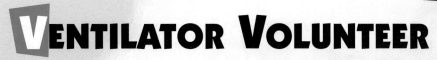

VENTILATOR VOLUNTEER

Preparation

1. Set up the mechanical ventilator.
2. Collect one endotracheal tube per volunteer.

Implementation

1. Distribute the endotracheal tube to each volunteer.
2. Ask volunteers to breathe through the end of the endotracheal tube for a few minutes and ask how they feel.
3. Connect the ventilator to the end of the endotracheal tube giving each volunteer a turn.
4. Demonstrate different modes of ventilation as well as flow synchronization.
5. Ask the volunteers how it felt using the various modes.
6. Use related graphics to illustrate points related to mechanical ventilation.

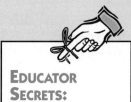

EDUCATOR
SECRETS:
This hands-on exercise
allows participants to
experience how a
patient feels on
mechanical ventilation.

By: Mary LaBiche, MEd, RRT

5-20 minutes

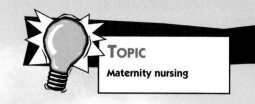

TOOL BOX

Markers, flip chart and easel or white board, index cards, timing device

COMMON DISCOMFORTS OF PREGNANCY

Preparation

1. Copy each item from Common Discomforts of Pregnancy on an index card.
2. Set up a flip chart and easel or white board and markers.
3. Obtain a timing device.

Implementation

1. Divide the group into two teams with an equal number of participants on each team.
2. Place Common Discomforts of Pregnancy index cards face down.
3. Explain the following rules:

   a. A team member will draw a Common Discomforts of Pregnancy card.

   b. The team member drawing the card reads it silently and draws on the flip chart or white board an illustration that will assist other team members in guessing the discomfort listed on the index card.

   c. There is no communication between the card holder and the team.

   d. The team is allowed one minute to guess what discomfort is on the card.

   e. The team must identify the appropriate nursing or medical interventions and teaching for each correct answer.

   f. A point is awarded for each correct answer.

   g. After one team completes their playing time, move to the next team.

   h. The team with the highest number of points wins.

EDUCATOR SECRETS:

Visual cues are a fun way to reinforce the knowledge of discomforts of pregnancy and treatments and interventions.

By: Chris Reed, RN, MSN
Bernadette Price, RN, MSN

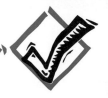

COMMON DISCOMFORTS OF PREGNANCY

Morning sickness

Headache

Constipation

Hemorrhoids

Leukorrhea

Ptyalism

Pyrosis

Fatigue

Chloasma

Palmar erythema

Gingivitis

Edema

Urinary frequency

Nasal stuffiness

Carpal tunnel syndrome

Insomnia

Mood swings

Backache

Linea nigra

Striae

Food cravings

Leg cramps

Varicosis

Syncope

Heart palpitations

Breast changes (enlargement, nipple changes)

Vena cava syndrome

20 minutes

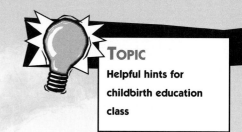
TOOL BOX

Childbirth Education Crossword Puzzle, Childbirth Education Crossword Puzzle Answer Key, pens or pencils

CHILDBIRTH EDUCATION CROSSWORD PUZZLE

Preparation

1. Copy the Childbirth Education Crossword Puzzle for each participant or labor team.

2. Use this as an introduction to the lesson or as a review after the lesson.

3. Copy the Childbirth Education Crossword Puzzle Answer Key.

4. Make sure all participants have a pen or pencil.

Variation

1. Use a poster printer copy machine to turn the crossword into a poster-size image.

2. Plan for groups of two to six to discuss and fill in the poster-size copy of the crossword puzzle before or after your lesson.

Implementation

1. Distribute Childbirth Education Crossword Puzzle sheet to each participant or labor team.

2. Challenge participants to complete the puzzle as individuals or as teams.

3. Share the correct answers as you desire.

Suggestion: The puzzle may also be sent out to reinforce learning days or weeks after the lesson.

EDUCATOR SECRETS:

If you have different ability levels in your session, pair learners of opposite abilities to maximize benefits to all.

By: Michele L. Deck, MEd, BSN, RN, ACCE-R

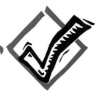

CHILDBIRTH EDUCATION CROSSWORD PUZZLE

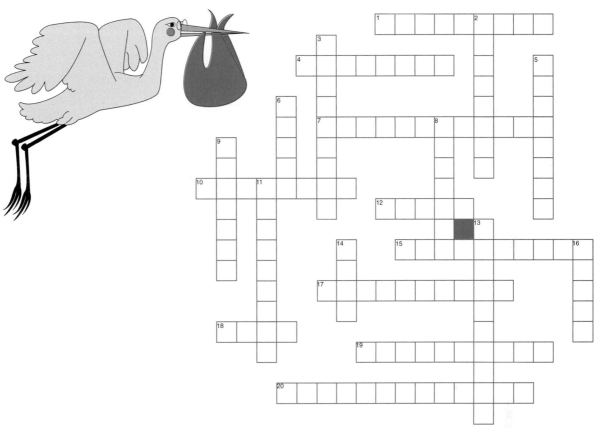

Across

1. This discharge is pearly, white, or pink in color before labor begins.

4. Call a professional caretaker when this breaks for further instruction.

7. The abdomen gets hard and then relaxes when these occur.

10. This structure provides oxygen and nutrients to the baby throughout pregnancy.

12. Go to the hospital if you have a teaspoon or more of this as a discharge before you deliver the baby.

15. This is another name for the placenta.

17. A woman focuses her eyes on this spot, object, or person to assist in concentration and relaxation.

18. This is the color babies become when they first cry heartily.

19. This incision is sometimes made to enlarge the perineal opening for delivery.

20. This is clamped and cut after the baby is born.

Down

2. Change this frequently when lying down in labor.

3. Place a cool, moistened one of these on the head or neck for comfort.

5. This is applied with the fist to the lower back for the relief of back labor.

6. Using this to talk to the baby will comfort and soothe the baby.

8. The labor support person will give this throughout labor and delivery.

9. This activity can enhance the strength of contractions.

11. This type of breath is good to take at the beginning and end of every contraction.

13. This is the most challenging time to keep the woman relaxed and comfortable.

14. When the woman first has the urge to push, she should do this instead until someone can check her progress.

16. A woman having a first baby will average 12 to 24 of these in labor.

161

CHILDBIRTH EDUCATION CROSSWORD PUZZLE

Answer Key

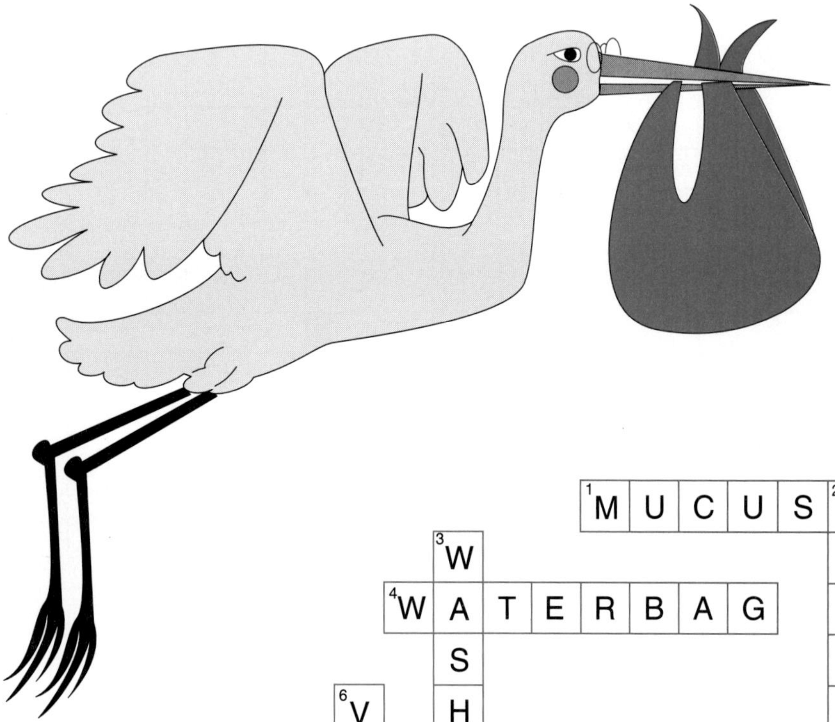

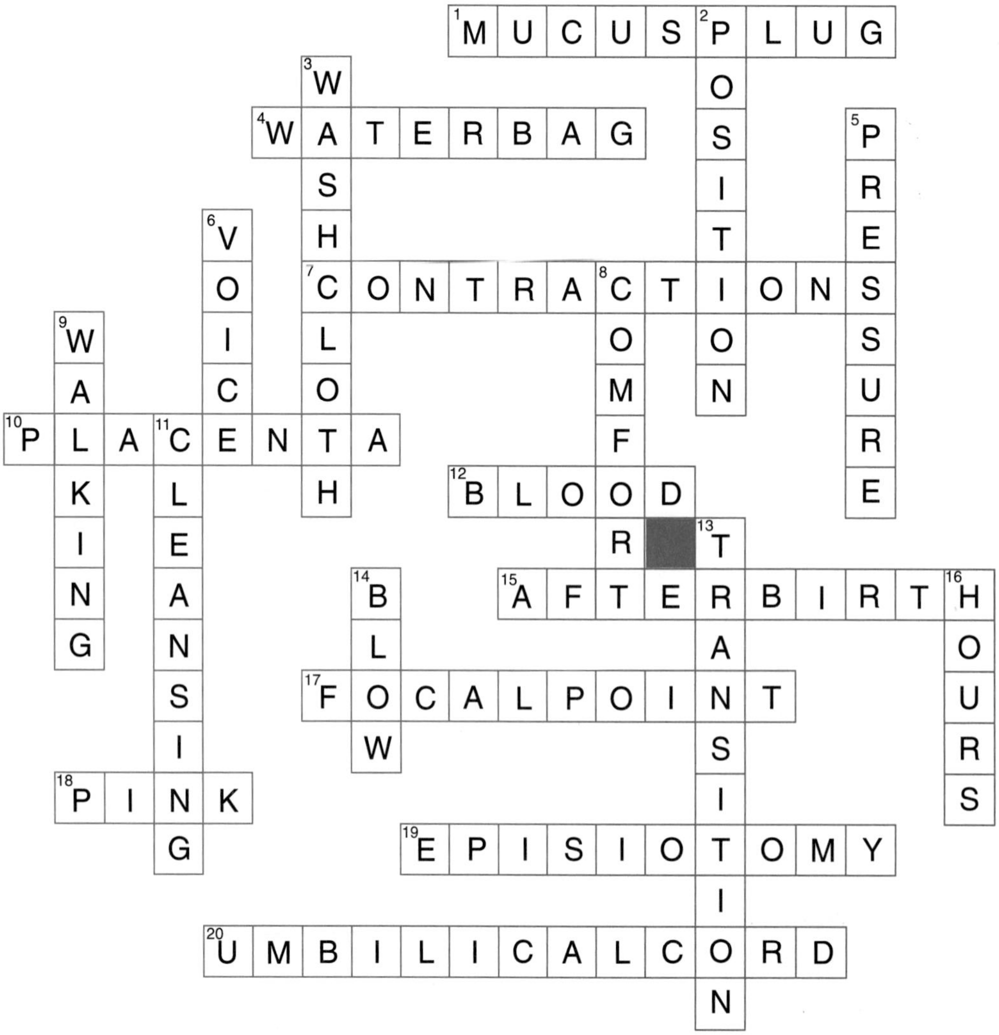
1 MUCUSPLUG
2 POSITION
3 WASHCLOTH
4 WATERBAG
5 PRESSURE
6 VOICE
7 CONTRACTIONS
8 COMFORT
9 WALKING
10 PLACENTA
11 CLEANSING
12 BLOOD
13 TRANSITION
14 BLOW
15 AFTERBIRTH
16 HOURS
17 FOCALPOINT
18 PINK
19 EPISIOTOMY
20 UMBILICALCORD

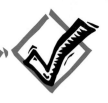

CHILDBIRTH EDUCATION CROSSWORD PUZZLE

Answer Key

Across

1. Mucus plug
4. Water bag
7. Contractions
10. Placenta
12. Blood
15. Afterbirth
17. Focal point
18. Pink
19. Episiotomy
20. Umbilical cord

Down

2. Position
3. Washcloth
5. Pressure
6. Voice
8. Comfort
9. Walking
11. Cleansing
13. Transition
14. Blow
16. Hours

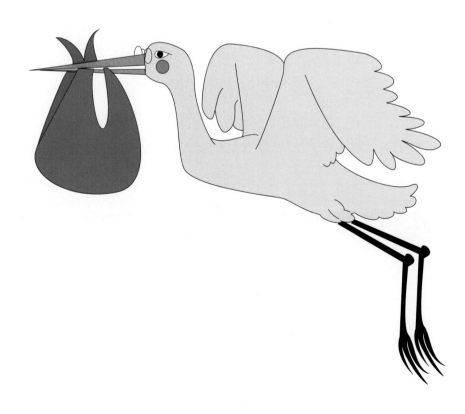

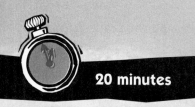

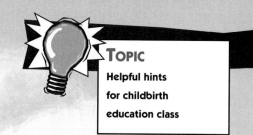

TOOL BOX

Childbirth Education
Fill-Ins, Childbirth
Education Answer Key,
pens or pencils

CHILDBIRTH EDUCATION FILL-INS

Preparation

1. Copy the Childbirth Education Fill-Ins for each participant or labor team.

2. Use this as an introduction to the lesson or as a review after the lesson.

3. Copy the Childbirth Education Answer Key.

4. Make sure all participants have a pen or pencil.

Variation: Use a poster printer copy machine to turn the Childbirth Education Fill-In into a poster-size image. Plan for groups of two to six to discuss and fill in the poster-size copy of the exercise before or after your lesson.

Implementation

1. Distribute a Childbirth Education Fill-In sheet to each participant or labor team.

2. Challenge participants to complete the sheet individually or in teams.

3. Explain to the participants that they are to fill in the blanks with the words supplied at the right side of the page. Once a word choice is made, it cannot be used again.

4. Share the correct answers as you desire.

Suggestion: Send out Childbirth Education Fill-Ins days or weeks after the class to reinforce learning.

EDUCATOR SECRETS:

Participants can work as
teams to answer the
questions to lower
anxiety and increase
learning.

By: Michele L. Deck, MEd,
BSN, RN, ACCE-R

164

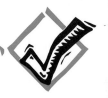

CHILDBIRTH EDUCATION FILL-INS

Directions: Fill in the blanks with the key terms. Each word can be used only once. Good Luck!

1. When the water bags leaks or _____ , call your professional labor support person for advice.

2. An average first labor can last approximately twelve to twenty-four _____ .

3. If you experience a _____ discharge at any point in pregnancy, call your professional labor support person.

4. _____ feel like a tightening of the abdomen.

5. The labor support person can suggest that the laboring woman change _____ when feeling discomfort.

6. Emptying the bladder can _____ pressure in the lower abdomen.

7. Progressive _____ can increase the comfort of the laboring woman.

8. A focal _____ is an internal or external visual to assist the woman to focus during contractions.

9. The labor support person has a time _____ the laboring woman does not have.

10. Encourage the woman to take contractions _____ at a time.

11. Light-touch massage, also known as _____ , can block sensation at the level of the skin.

12. The _____ provides oxygen and nutrients to the baby in utero.

13. It is important to keep the baby _____ when first delivered because the baby must learn to adjust his or her own body temperature.

14. _____ is the most challenging time to keep a woman without anesthesia calm in labor.

15. Pushing the baby out is hard but _____ work.

16. A deep _____ breath can be an oxygen boost at the beginning and end of a contraction.

17. Massage can work to _____ women in labor.

18. A _____ delivery is a surgical delivery of the baby.

19. The newborn baby can recognize sounds and _____ .

20. After the baby is born, a woman will have a vaginal _____ .

Key Terms

discharge

cleansing

placenta

point

breaks

voices

rewarding

effleurage

relaxation

hours

cesarean

transition

one

decrease

bloody

relax

warm

perspective

positions

contractions

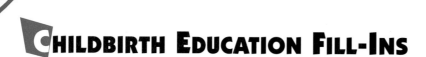

CHILDBIRTH EDUCATION FILL-INS

Answer Key

1. When the water bags leaks or **breaks**, call your professional labor support person for advice.

2. An average first labor can last approximately twelve to twenty-four **hours**.

3. If you experience a **bloody** discharge at any point in pregnancy, call your professional labor support person.

4. **Contractions** feel like a tightening of the abdomen.

5. The labor support person can suggest that the laboring woman change **positions** when feeling discomfort.

6. Emptying the bladder can **decrease** pressure in the lower abdomen.

7. Progressive **relaxation** can increase the comfort of the laboring woman.

8. A focal **point** is an internal or external visual to assist the woman to focus during contractions.

9. The labor support person has a time **perspective** the laboring woman does not have.

10. Encourage the woman to take contractions **one** at a time.

11. Light-touch massage, also known as **effleurage**, can block sensation at the level of the skin.

12. The **placenta** provides oxygen and nutrients to the baby in utero.

13. It is important to keep the baby **warm** when first delivered because the baby must learn to adjust his or her own body temperature.

14. **Transition** is the most challenging time to keep a woman without anesthesia calm in labor.

15. Pushing the baby out is hard but **rewarding** work.

16. A deep **cleansing** breath can be an oxygen boost at the beginning and end of a contraction.

17. Massage can work to **relax** women in labor.

18. A **cesarean** delivery is a surgical delivery of the baby.

19. The newborn baby can recognize sounds and **voices**.

20. After the baby is born, a woman will have a vaginal **discharge**.

ABG Go Fish

Preparation

1. Determine the number of participants and divide into teams of four participants.

2. Obtain envelopes, one for each team.

3. Obtain index cards or colored paper in two different colors.

4. Make an ABG Go Fish card set (set includes parameters and analysis) for each team using the following guidelines:

   If you choose to use colored index cards:

   a. Copy the ABG Go Fish Parameters and Analysis sheets for each team.

   b. Cut out each parameter and paste it to one color (such as yellow) index card.

   c. Cut out each analysis and paste it to a different color (such as blue) index card.

   If you choose colored paper:

   a. Copy the ABG Go Fish Parameters on colored paper (such as yellow), one sheet per team.

   b. Copy the ABG Go Fish Analysis on a different color paper (such as blue), one sheet per team.

   c. Cut out one Parameter sheet and one Analysis sheet for each team.

5. Place each set (yellow and blue) in an envelope, one set per envelope and one envelope per team.

Implementation

1. Divide participants into teams of four.

2. Create pairs within each team of four. Call one pair 1 and the other pair 2.

3. Distribute an envelope to each team of four participants.

4. Ask the teams to empty their envelope and place all cards face down.

By: Sandy Woodbury, RN, MS, CCRN

continued

ABC Go Fish *continued*

5. Provide the following directions:

   a. Yellow cards contain parameters and blue cards contain analysis.

   b. One of the 1's will start the play by turning over one of each color card.

   c. 1's discuss if the parameter and analysis match. The pair must agree it is a match to continue play.

   d. If both 1's agree it is a match, they consult with the 2's on the team to reach consensus. The team must agree the cards match.

   e. If a match is made, the two cards are removed from the card group and placed in front of the pair who made the match. A point is recorded for the match.

   f. If a match is not made, the cards return to play and are placed face down.

6. Play alternates between pairs within a team until all the analysis and parameter cards are matched.

7. Award the pair with the most points a small prize.

ABC Go Fish

Parameters

Directions: Copy and cut out boxes.

Metabolic acidosis

Respiratory alkalosis, compensated

Respiratory alkalosis

Metabolic acidosis, compensated

Metabolic alkalosis

Respiratory alkalosis

Respiratory acidosis, partially compensated

Metabolic acidosis

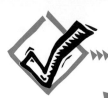

ABC Go Fish

Analysis

Directions: Copy and cut out boxes.

pH 7.05
PCO_2 12
HCO_3 5

pH 7.48
PCO_2 42
HCO_3 30

pH 7.37
PCO_2 25
HCO_3 14

pH 7.54
PCO_2 26
HCO_3 22

pH 7.33
PCO_2 34
HCO_3 16.6

pH 7.41
PCO_2 25
HCO_3 15

pH 7.34
PCO_2 60
HCO_3 34

pH 7.48
PCO_2 22
HCO_3 17

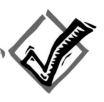

ABC Go Fish

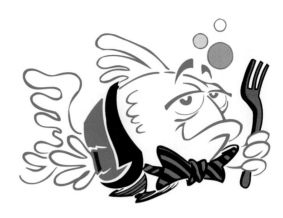

Answer Key

Metabolic acidosis	pH 7.33 PCO_2 34 HCO_3 16.6
Metabolic alkalosis	pH 7.48 PCO_2 42 HCO_3 30
Respiratory alkalosis	pH 7.54 PCO_2 26 HCO_3 22
Respiratory acidosis, partially compensated	pH 7.34 PCO_2 60 CO_3 34
Respiratory alkalosis, compensated	pH 7.41 PCO_2 25 HCO_3 15
Respiratory alkalosis	pH 7.48 PCO_2 22 HCO_3 17
Metabolic acidosis	pH 7.05 PCO_2 12 HCO_3 5
Metabolic acidosis, compensated	pH 7.37 PCO_2 25 HCO_3 14

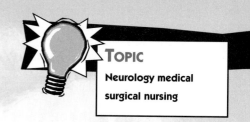
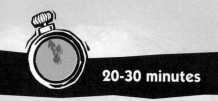
20-30 minutes

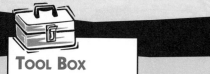

NEURO CELEBRITY SQUARES

Preparation

1. Copy the Neuro Celebrity Squares Questions and Answers sheet, or create your own questions and answers.

2. Place four to five chairs in front of the room close to the white board or flip chart (panelist seating).

3. Obtain markers.

4. Provide prizes.

Implementation

1. Recruit or select four to five volunteers to be panelists.

2. Appoint one panelist to be the recorder.

3. Have one panelist draw a tic-tac-toe grid on the white board or flip chart large enough for all to see.

4. Divide the remaining class members into two groups, one group of X's and one group of O's.

5. Invite one participant from the O's and one participant from the X's to act as spokespersons for their groups.

6. Select a team to be first and ask the team's spokesperson a question from the Neuro Celebrity Squares Questions and Answers sheet.

7. Provide the following instructions:

   a. The team spokesperson selects one of the panelists to answer the question.

   b. The panelist can bluff or answer correctly.

   c. The team advises the spokesperson on whether to agree or disagree with the panelist's answer.

continued

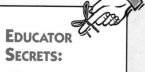

By: Nancy Moulaison, RN, BSN

NEURO CELEBRITY SQUARES *continued*

d. The team spokesperson advises the facilitator if the team is in agreement or disagreement with the answer provided by the panelist.

e. If the answer the panelist gives is correct and the team agrees, an *X* or *O* (depending on the team) is marked on the tic-tac-toe grid and a point is scored.

f. If the answer the panelist gives is correct and the team agrees that the answer is incorrect, no mark is made on the tic-tac-toe grid and no points are scored.

g. If the answer the panelist gives is incorrect and the team notes the answer is incorrect (that is, disagrees with the panelist) their mark is made on the tic-tac-toe grid and a point is scored.

h. If the answer the panelist gives is incorrect and the team agrees it is the correct answer, no mark is made on the tic-tac-toe grid and no points are scored.

8. Play continues until one team completes a row of three marks on the tic-tac-toe grid.

9. Award small prizes to all.

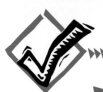

NEURO CELEBRITY SQUARES

Questions and Answers

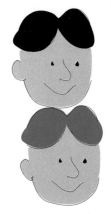

1. What is the difference between expressive and receptive aphasia?
   Answer: *With expressive aphasia, the person cannot speak well (the words are jumbled or incorrect). With receptive aphasia, the person cannot understand the spoken word.*

2. How do vital signs (blood pressure, pulse, and respiration) differ between shock and increased intracranial pressure?
   Answer: *Vital signs for shock are low blood pressure, high pulse, and high respiration. Vital signs for increased intracranial pressure are high blood pressure, low pulse, and irregular respiration.*

3. Describe the difference between hemiplegia and paraplegia.
   Answer: *Hemiplegia involves paralysis of one-half of the body, from head down to the feet on the affected side. Paraplegia involves paralysis of both legs.*

4. Describe hemianopsia.
   Answer: *Hemianopsia occurs after a CVA where the patient loses one-half of the vision of each eye; the loss occurs on the side of the CVA.*

5. What does the word *dysphagia* mean?
   Answer: Dysphagia *means difficulty swallowing.*

6. What is the medical abbreviation for "little stroke?"
   Answer: *The medical abbreviation used is T. I. A.*

7. Who has more CVAs, men or women?
   Answer: *Men have more CVAs than women.*

8. What is a cerebral embolus?
   Answer: *A cerebral embolus is a clot that has traveled from another part of the body and has lodged in the brain (cerebral artery).*

9. Relating to CVAs, what is primitive speech?
   Answer: *Primitive speech is the basic speech pattern in which the CVA patient recites poems or words over and over or counts a few numbers over and over.*

10. What is an aura?
    Answer: *An aura is a warning of impending seizure. Usually the patient sees flashing lights or vision becomes super clear.*

11. What is the Glasgow scale used for?
    Answer: *The Glasgow coma scale is used to determine level of coma.*

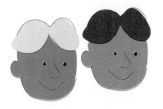

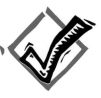

NEURO CELEBRITY SQUARES

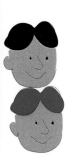

12. Describe trigeminal neuralgia.
Which cranial nerve is involved?
Answer: *Trigeminal neuralgia is an inflammation of the fifth cranial nerve involving severe spasms of facial pain.*

13. How many cranial nerves are there?
Answer: *There are 12 cranial nerves.*

14. Name the first cranial nerve.
Answer: *The first cranial nerve is the olfactory.*

15. Name two drugs used to treat seizures.
Answer: *Drugs used to treat seizures include: Tegretol, phenobarbitol, Valium, Dilantin, and Klonopin.*

16. Name the three layers of the meninges covering the brain and spinal cord.
Answer: *Layers of the meninges include the dura mater, arachnoid, and pia mater.*

17. What is the most common patient complaint after a spinal tap is done?
Answer: *The most common complaint after a spinal tap is a headache.*

18. What is the difference between a convulsion and a seizure?
Answer: *A convulsion is the tonic/clonic twitching, jerking motion. A seizure encompasses the whole episode from aura to convulsion to postictal sleep.*

19. Name the seventh cranial nerve.
Answer: *The seventh cranial nerve is the facial nerve.*

20. Where in the spinal column does the spinal cord end? Be specific.
Answer: *The spinal cord ends just below lumbar one vertebrae.*

21. Is the autonomic nervous system part of the central nervous system or the peripheral nervous system?
Answer: *The autonomic nervous system is part of the peripheral nervous system.*

22. What sound does the physician have the patient make when checking the twelfth cranial nerve?
Answer: *The physician has the patient make the "la, la, la, la" sound.*

NEURO CELEBRITY SQUARES

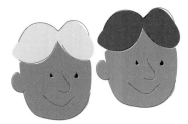

23. Which division of the autonomic nervous system is our "fight or flight" system?
    Answer: *Our "fight or flight" system is the sympathetic nervous system.*

24. Which system of the autonomic nervous system is our "settle down" system?
    Answer: *Our parasympathetic system is our "settle down" system.*

25. What do the letters L. O. C. mean in the medical community?
    Answer: *L. O. C. means level of consciousness.*

26. What is the difference between the tonic phase and clonic phase of a convulsion?
    Answer: *The tonic phase of a convulsion is the teeth clenching, body stiffening part; the clonic phase is the jerking, thrashing part of the convulsion.*

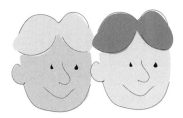

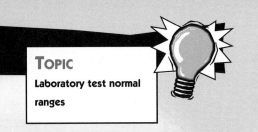

15 minutes

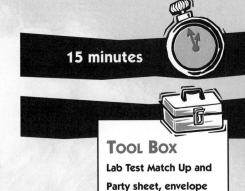

TOOL BOX
Lab Test Match Up and Party sheet, envelope or container with lid

LAB TEST MATCH UP AND PARTY

Preparation

1. Make two copies of the Lab Test Match Up and Party sheets. Keep one intact to use as an answer key.

2. Cut out boxes along the solid lines and paste to thin cardboard to make cards.

3. Cut cards along the perforated lines.

4. Store cards in envelope or container with lid.

Implementation

1. Walk around the room and have each participant pick out one item from the envelope/container.

2. Allow five to ten minutes for participants to get up and find the participant that holds the match to make a complete card. Once everyone has found their match, the pair works together to look up two to three facts about that lab test.

3. Call time when all are ready.

4. Have each pair read aloud the lab test, the normal range, and two or three facts about the test.

Suggestion: If you have more participants than lab tests, make duplicate sets.

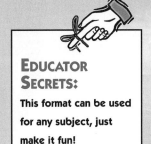

EDUCATOR SECRETS:
This format can be used for any subject, just make it fun!

By: Nancy Moulaison, RN, BSN

177

Lab Test Match Up and Party

Directions: Copy and cut apart on lines. Retain an extra copy for an answer key.

Blood urea nitrogen

Serum normal range 10-20 mg/dl

Sodium

Serum normal range 135-145 Meq/L

Potassium

Serum normal range 3.5-5.5 Meq/L

Blood glucose

Serum normal range 80-120 mg/dl

Hematocrit

Serum normal
Males 42%-52%
Females 37%-47%

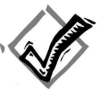

LAB TEST MATCH UP AND PARTY

Directions: Copy and cut apart on lines. Retain an extra copy for an answer key.

Hemoglobin

Serum normal
Males 14-18 gms/dl
Females 12-16 gms/dl

White blood
count

Serum normal
range
5000-10,000/mm^3

Red blood
count

Serum
normal range
4.5-5.5 million/mm^3
of blood

Platelets

Serum
normal range
150,0000-
400,000/mm^3 of blood

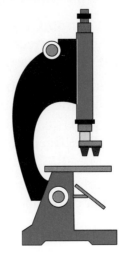

15 minutes

TOOL BOX

Jumpin' Jamboree
Challenge Questions,
Not Answers; Jumpin'
Jamboree Challenge
Answer Key;
transparency; overhead
projector; Post-it™ notes

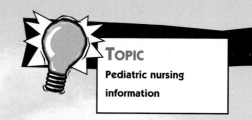

TOPIC
Pediatric nursing
information

JUMPIN' JAMBOREE CHALLENGE QUESTIONS, NOT ANSWERS

Preparation

1. Copy the Jumpin' Jamboree Challenge Questions, Not Answers, onto an overhead transparency.

2. Obtain Post-it™ notes and cover each square on the Jumpin' Jamboree Challenge Questions, Not Answers transparency with a Post-it™ note.

3. Copy the Jumpin' Jamboree Challenge Answer Key.

Implementation

1. Divide the group into two teams to compete against each other.

2. Select a team leader for each team.

3. Show Jumpin' Jamboree Challenge Questions, Not Answers (with the squares covered) on an overhead projector.

4. Pick a team to go first.

5. Have the team leader pick a category.

6. Remove Post-it™ notes as a category is selected, and announce the statement and amount to the group.

7. Allow the first person on the team to "jump up," after the complete statement is read, to state the appropriate question (the answer stated as a question).

8. Award and record the designated points if the question is correct. If the question is incorrect, anyone on the opposing team can jump up and state their question. If the stated question is correct, that team receives the point and the opportunity to pick a category.

9. Award small prizes or bragging rights to the team scoring the highest number of points.

EDUCATOR SECRETS:

The jumpin' adds energy and fun to the activity!

By: Kathy Harding, MSN, RN

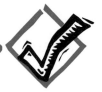

JUMPIN' JAMBOREE CHALLENGE QUESTIONS, NOT ANSWERS

State the question that matches the answer.

Take Out	Measure Up	Safety First	Ivy League	Play Time
1 The initials I and O stand for this.	**1** One ounce equals this many cc's.	**1** You always keep these up.	**1** You should keep two hours' worth of fluid in this.	**1** This is a very important part of pediatrics.
2 Intake and output evaluate this.	**2** One grain equals this many mg's.	**2** This should be in the lowest position.	**2** You need to keep this closed and the air vent open.	**2** Babies handle stress by this activity.
3 Urine output is measured in these.	**3** 1 gram equals this many mg's.	**3** It is important to check that these are up.	**3** This should be assessed every two hours.	**3** A good nurse picks this type of toy for each patient.
4 One gram of urine equals this many cc's.	**4** 1 tsp. equals this many cc's.	**4** This piece of equipment should be in reach of the parent and patient.	**4** Press this button on the IVAC to find the total at 6 P.M.	**4** Children believe in this.
5 On pedi the I/O is recorded at this time.	**5** 1 kg equals this many lbs.	**5** Be sure to have this on a child when in the high chair.	**5** This is used to cover the IV site.	**5** Children are these two types of thinkers.

JUMPIN' JAMBOREE CHALLENGE QUESTIONS, NOT ANSWERS

Answer Key

Take Out	Measure Up	Safety First	Ivy League	Play Time
1 What is intake and output?	1 What is 30 cc?	1 What are side rails?	1 What is a Buretrol?	1 What is play therapy?
2 What is hydration?	2 What is 60 mg?	2 What is the bed?	2 What is a safety clamp?	2 What is sucking?
3 What are cc's?	3 What is 1000 mg?	3 What are side rails?	3 What is the IV site and rate?	3 What is age appropriate?
4 What is 1 cc?	4 What is 5 cc?	4 What is the call bell?	4 What is volume infused?	4 What is magic?
5 What is 6 P.M.?	5 What is 2.21 lbs?	5 What is a seat belt restraint?	5 What is a stockinette?	5 What is magical or concrete?

TOOL BOX

Stethoscopes, ear plugs, cotton balls, radio or musical tuner, glasses or sunglasses, petroleum jelly or lotion, gag glasses, gloves, popsicle sticks, tape, medicine bottles with childproof caps, multiple medications, white pills, seven-day medicine dispenser, medic alert tags, cane, splints, robe, sweater, slippers

GERIATRICS REALITY CHECK

Preparation

1. Assemble all Tool Box equipment in a large shopping bag.

2. Prepare geriatric content for your presentation, and identify key learning points.

3. Select your geriatric wardrobe—robe, slippers, sweater, sweatshirt, gag glasses, cane, etc.

4. Ready audio equipment.

5. Place an assortment of "white" over the counter pills in the seven-day container.

6. Glue popsicle sticks parallel to glove fingers (to demonstrate accomplishing a daily task with rigid fingers).

7. Rub glasses with petroleum jelly or lotion.

Implementation

1. Walk into your class using a cane and wearing the robe, slippers, sweater, sweatshirt, and gag glasses.

2. Ask the class to describe the stereotype of the geriatric patient.

3. Distribute stethoscopes, ear plugs, and cotton balls, and ask participants to place the item they have been handed in their ears.

4. Turn on the radio and set between frequencies to generate static and simulate background noise, or set music tuner to a high frequency to simulate tinnitus (a common side-effect of several medications used in the elderly population).

5. Distribute glasses or sunglasses smeared with petroleum jelly or lotion to simulate visual changes of glaucoma and cataracts.

6. Pass out gloves with popsicle sticks attached and the childproof medicine bottles and ask the participants to write and open the medicine bottles. This exercise simulates limited dexterity caused by arthritis.

continued

EDUCATOR SECRETS:

Participants have a better appreciation for elderly patients after they become one, because of their personal experience. Add the element of surprise and instant attention by coming into the class in your "costume" a few minutes late so that all participants are seated.

By: Janet Fitts, RN, BSN, CEN, TNS, EMT-P

GERIATRICS REALITY CHECK *continued*

7. Pass out the seven-day pill container (containing all white pills), and ask participants to determine what each pill is, and whether or not it appears to be a prescription medication. (This exercise illustrates some of the problems with polypharmacy in the elderly.)

8. Discuss stereotyping in the elderly.

9. Ask a willing participant to perform the interview portion of a routine assessment with you as the geriatric patient. When asked for medication, give the participant the brown paper bag that has only loose medications left in it.

10. Begin a discussion on medication use in the elderly.

11. Ask the participants to put on their elderly props and present information for five to ten minutes.

12. Stop and ask the participants to describe what it felt like to experience first-hand the limitations of the elderly.

ACUTE RENAL FAILURE WORD SEARCH

TOOL BOX

Acute Renal Failure
Word Search puzzle,
Acute Renal Failure
Word Search Answer
Key transparency,
overhead projector,
pens or pencils, small
prizes (optional)

Preparation

1. Make a copy of Acute Renal Failure Word Search puzzle for each participant.

2. Copy Acute Renal Failure Word Search Answer Key onto an overhead transparency.

3. Set up the overhead projector.

4. Make sure that each participant has a pencil or pen.

5. Obtain small prizes (optional).

Implementation

1. Distribute the Acute Renal Failure Word Search puzzle to each participant.

2. Challenge your learners to complete the fill-in-the-blank questions.

3. Encourage the participants to use the lecture notes to help them with tough answers.

4. Invite the participants to search for the answers in the Word Search puzzle sheet.

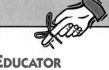

EDUCATOR SECRETS:

The puzzle can be used for content review after a lecture or sent out days or weeks later.

By: Jana Magarelli, RN, MA

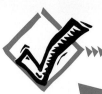

ACUTE RENAL FAILURE WORD SEARCH

Directions: Answer the fill-in-the-blank questions and complete the puzzle using the answers. Good luck!

A. Acute renal failure is classified in three categories: (1) _____ , (2) _____ , and (3) _____ .

B. There are three phases in the cycle of acute tubular necrosis: (4) _____ phase, (5) _____ phase, and (6) _____ phase.

C. Approximately 50% of acute renal failure patients produce urine. Therefore, urine volume alone is not an adequate guide to renal function. Progressive (7) _____ occurs as a result of decreased glomerular filtration rate in spite of apparently adequate urine output.

D. Medullary involvement of the kidneys specifically affects the (8) _____ portions of the nephrons, causing (9) _____ .

E. There are four major problems of patient care in acute renal failure: (10) _____ , (11) _____ , (12) _____ , and (13) _____ .

```
L  I  N  C  R  E  A  S  E  C  A  T  A  B  O  L  I  S  M  S
O  I  F  L  U  I  D  O  V  E  R  L  O  A  D  Z  Y  Q  Y  Z
V  N  D  U  R  G  P  H  P  A  P  I  E  N  S  W  R  O  I  U
E  T  L  M  N  O  R  F  A  I  R  W  A  T  O  P  A  F  N  O
S  R  E  C  O  V  E  R  Y  P  A  M  C  R  E  A  L  I  F  P
C  A  I  N  C  A  R  D  U  E  C  A  T  I  O  N  U  O  E  I
N  R  L  A  T  H  E  P  O  S  T  R  E  N  A  L  B  L  C  I
J  E  M  U  S  E  N  K  Y  E  N  T  U  E  G  O  U  I  T  M
A  N  C  X  Y  Z  A  Z  O  T  E  M  I  A  B  N  T  G  I  N
S  A  A  R  B  C  L  J  I  K  L  W  P  Q  V  M  G  U  O  A
M  L  D  E  O  F  I  N  T  R  A  R  E  N  A  L  S  R  N  M
I  M  E  S  A  S  B  V  G  O  U  T  F  E  I  L  T  I  D  C
N  P  A  N  D  E  I  R  U  Q  D  I  U  R  E  T  I  C  P  L
E  L  A  N  C  E  T  S  R  E  A  B  B  I  S  E  W  F  Y  Q
E  L  E  C  T  R  O  L  Y  T  E  I  M  B  A  L  A  N  C  E
```

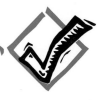

ACUTE RENAL FAILURE WORD SEARCH

Answer Key

A. Acute renal failure is classified in three categories: (1) **prerenal**, (2) **intrarenal**, and (3) **postrenal**.

B. There are three phases in the cycle of acute tubular necrosis: (4) **oliguric** phase, (5) **diuretic** phase, and (6) **recovery** phase.

C. Approximately 50% of acute renal failure patients produce urine. Therefore urine volume alone is not an adequate guide to renal function. Progressive (7) **azotemia** occurs as a result of decreased glomerular filtration rate in spite of apparently adequate urine output.

D. Medullary involvement of the kidneys specifically affects the (8) **tubular** portions of the nephrons, causing (9) **necrosis**.

E. There are four major problems of patient care in acute renal failure: (10) **infection**, (11) **increase catabolism**, (12) **electrolyte imbalance**, and (13) **fluid overload**.

```
L   I   N   C   R   E   A   S   E   C   A   T   A   B   O   L   I   S   M   S
O   I   F   L   U   I   D   O   V   E   R   L   O   A   D   Z   Y   Q   Y   Z
V   N   D   U   R   G   P   H   P   A   P   I   E   N   S   W   R   O   I   U
E   T   L   M   N   O   R   F   A   I   R   W   A   T   O   P   A   F   N   O
S   R   E   C   O   V   E   R   Y   P   A   M   C   R   E   A   L   I   F   P
C   A   I   N   C   A   R   D   U   E   C   A   T   I   O   N   U   O   E   I
N   R   L   A   T   H   E   P   O   S   T   R   E   N   A   L   B   L   C   I
J   E   M   U   S   E   N   K   Y   E   N   T   U   E   G   O   U   I   T   M
A   N   C   X   Y   Z   A   Z   O   T   E   M   I   A   B   N   T   G   I   N
S   A   A   R   B   C   L   J   I   K   L   W   P   Q   V   M   G   U   O   A
M   L   D   E   O   F   I   N   T   R   A   R   E   N   A   L   S   R   N   M
I   M   E   S   A   S   B   V   G   O   U   T   F   E   I   L   T   I   D   C
N   P   A   N   D   E   I   R   U   Q   D   I   U   R   E   T   I   C   P   L
E   L   A   N   C   E   T   S   R   E   A   B   B   I   S   E   W   F   Y   Q
E   L   E   C   T   R   O   L   Y   T   E   I   M   B   A   L   A   N   C   E
```

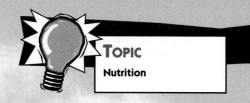

TOPIC
Nutrition

TOOL BOX

Food for Thought
sheets and Answer Key
sheet; beans or pencils,
pens, or markers; small
prizes (optional)

FOOD FOR THOUGHT

Preparation

1. Make a copy of Food for Thought for each participant.

2. Copy the Food for Thought Answer Key.

3. Provide beans to be used as card covers, or pens, pencils, or markers.

4. Obtain small prizes (optional).

Implementation

1. Distribute a Food for Thought sheet to each participant.

2. Distribute beans or a pen, pencil, or marker to each participant.

3. Explain that you will read a statement and participants are to mark the answer on the Food for Thought sheet.

4. Invite the participants to call out "Foodo" when their card is completely covered.

5. Use the Food for Thought Answer Key to check answers.
   NOTE: There are two correct answers for some statements.

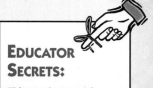

EDUCATOR SECRETS:

This can be used for
content preview or
review after a lecture.

By: Sandra H. Clark, MSN, RN

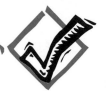

FOOD FOR THOUGHT

F	O	O	D	O
Corn on the cob	Liver	Orange juice	Vodka	Bananas
Cheddar cheese	Coffee	Cranberry juice	Milk	Saltines
Snickers bar	Oysters	Sweet lemonade	Cabbage	Salmon
Cucumbers	Carrots	Pickle juice	Bran cereal	Gatorade
Orange juice	Yogurt	Potato chips	Fried chicken	Dark green vegetables

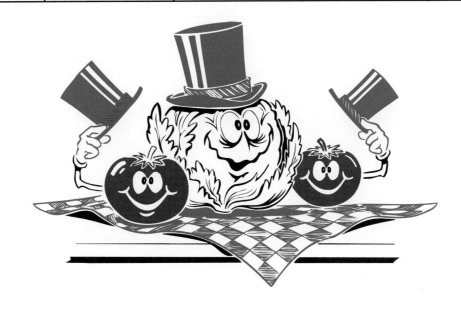

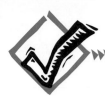

FOOD FOR THOUGHT

F	O	O	D	O
Liver	Oysters	Corn on the cob	Coffee	Cabbage
Cheddar cheese	Saltines	Salmon	Snickers bar	Gatorade
Yogurt	Cranberry juice	Saltines	Milk	Sweet lemonade
Cucumbers	Pickle juice	Carrots	Bran cereal	Vodka
Fried chicken	Bananas	Dark green vegetables	Orange juice	Potato chips

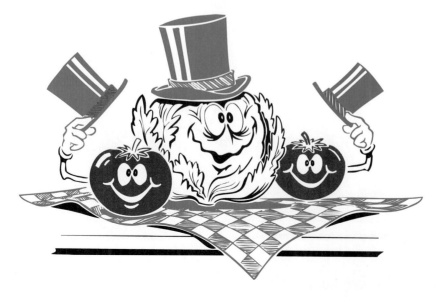

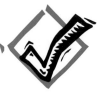

FOOD FOR THOUGHT

F	O	O	D	O
Milk	Oysters	Corn on the cob	Liver	Coffee
Cheddar cheese	Saltines	Salmon	Snickers bar	Gatorade
Bananas	Cranberry juice	Saltines	Cabbage	Sweet lemonade
Cucumbers	Carrots	Pickle juice	Bran cereal	Vodka
Fried chicken	Yogurt	Dark green vegetables	Orange juice	Potato chips

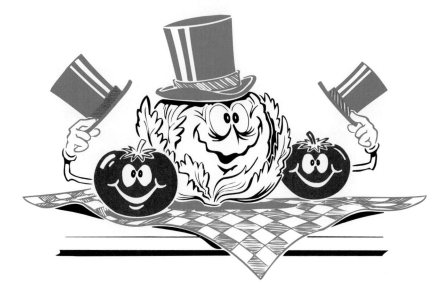

FOOD FOR THOUGHT

Answer Key

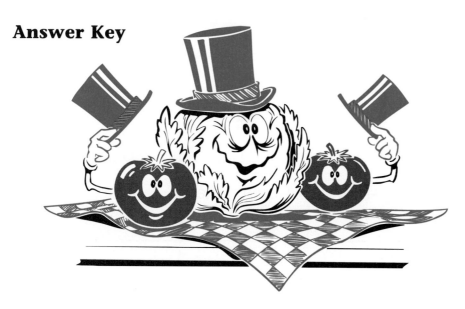

1.	Causes inflammation and destruction of pancreatic tissue.	Vodka
2.	Increases stool odor and intestinal gas.	Cabbage
3.	Avoid this in diverticulitis.	Corn on the cob
4.	Not enough contributes to rickets.	Milk or salmon
5.	Contributes to raising urine pH.	Orange juice
6.	Great source of potassium.	Bananas
7.	Could contribute to hypertension.	Potato chips or saltines
8.	Avoid this with the dumping syndrome.	Sweet lemonade
9.	Excellent to replace electrolytes.	Gatorade
10.	Helps to restore normal flora.	Yogurt
11.	May play a part in hepatitis.	Oysters
12.	Do not eat while taking MAO inhibitors.	Cheddar cheese
13.	May cause biliary colic.	Fried chicken
14.	Used to treat diverticulosis.	Bran cereal
15.	Deficiency may lead to osteoporosis.	Salmon or milk
16.	Neutralizes bases.	Pickle juice
17.	Used to decrease cholesterol.	Bran cereal
18.	Can be used to treat nausea.	Saltines or gatorade
19.	Produces symptoms similar to theophylline.	Coffee
20.	Inappropriate for gouty arthritis.	Liver
21.	Not included on a diabetic diet.	Snickers bar or sweet lemonade
22.	A free food.	Cucumbers
23.	Use carefully while on Coumadin.	Green vegetables or liver
24.	Great source of vitamin A.	Carrots
25.	Contributes to urine acidity.	Cranberry juice

TOPIC
**Home care orientation
for professional staff**

NAVIGATING THE HIM-11

TOOL BOX

Navigating the HIM-11
(Health Insurance
Manual, publication 11)
sheet, transparency,
overhead projector,
pens, or pencils.

Preparation

1. Make a copy of Navigating the HIM-11 [Publication 11 from Health Care Financing Administration (HCFA)] for each participant.

2. Make an overhead transparency of Navigating the HIM-11.

3. Set up the overhead projector.

4. Assure that each participant has a pencil or pen to take notes if desired.

Implementation

1. Distribute the Navigating the HIM-11 sheet to each participant.

2. Assure that each person has a pen or pencil to take additional notes as desired.

3. Explain that documentation plays a critical role in professional home care.

4. Stress the importance that clinicians know and understand the regulations to which they must adhere.

5. Show the Navigating the HIM-11 transparency on the overhead projector.

6. Explain and clarify each numbered cloud. For example, cloud 2 Homebound means it requires a considerable and taxing effort for the patient to leave home infrequently and for short durations.

**EDUCATOR
SECRETS:**

Using a graphic outline
format allows staff to
visualize the specific
criteria to which they
must adhere.

By: Mary Arnone Cahoon, BS, RN
Original layout by Val Spaulding

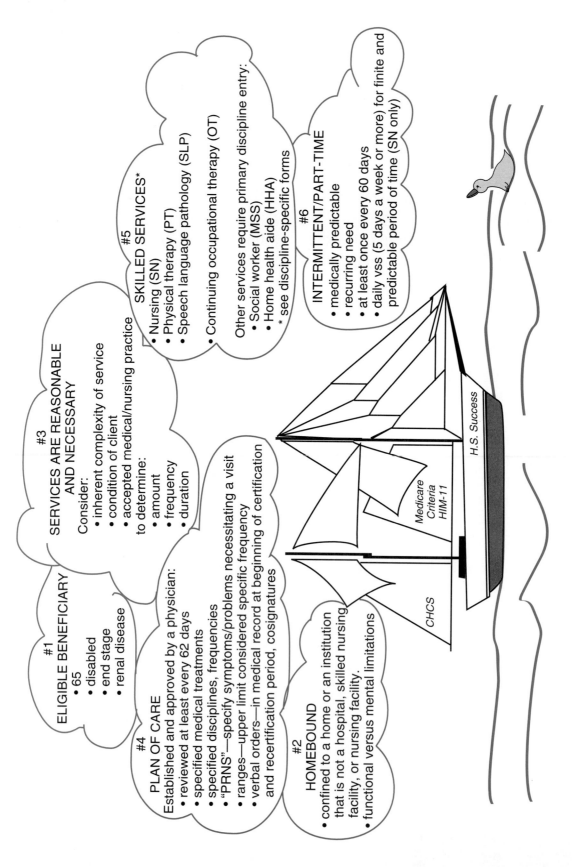

#3 SERVICES ARE REASONABLE AND NECESSARY
Consider:
- inherent complexity of service
- condition of client
- accepted medical/nursing practice

to determine:
- amount
- frequency
- duration

#5 SKILLED SERVICES*
- Nursing (SN)
- Physical therapy (PT)
- Speech language pathology (SLP)
- Continuing occupational therapy (OT)

Other services require primary discipline entry:
- Social worker (MSS)
- Home health aide (HHA)
- * see discipline-specific forms

#6 INTERMITTENT/PART-TIME
- medically predictable
- recurring need
- at least once every 60 days
- daily vss (5 days a week or more) for finite and predictable period of time (SN only)

#1 ELIGIBLE BENEFICIARY
- 65
- disabled
- end stage
- renal disease

#4 PLAN OF CARE
Established and approved by a physician:
- reviewed at least every 62 days
- specified medical treatments
- specified disciplines, frequencies
- "PRNS"—specify symptoms/problems necessitating a visit
- ranges—upper limit considered specific frequency
- verbal orders—in medical record at beginning of certification and recertification period, cosignatures

#2 HOMEBOUND
- confined to a home or an institution that is not a hospital, skilled nursing facility, or nursing facility.
- functional versus mental limitations

H.S. Success

Medicare Criteria HIM-11

CHCS

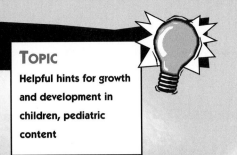
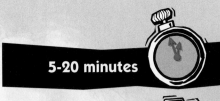

5-20 minutes

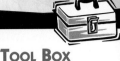

TOOL BOX

Looking Up . . .
A Child's View
Crossword Puzzle,
Looking Up . . .
A Child's View
Crossword Puzzle
Answer Key, pens
or pencils

LOOKING UP . . . A CHILD'S VIEW CROSSWORD PUZZLE

Preparation

1. Copy the Looking Up . . . A Child's View Crossword Puzzle for each participant.
2. Use this as an introduction to the lesson or as a review after the lesson.
3. Copy the Looking Up . . . A Child's View Crossword Puzzle Answer Key.
4. Make sure all participants have a pen or pencil.

Variation: Use a poster printer copy machine to turn the crossword into a poster-size image. Plan for groups of two to six to discuss and fill in the poster-size copy of the crossword puzzle before or after your lesson.

Implementation

1. Distribute the Looking Up . . . A Child's View Crossword Puzzle sheet to each participant.
2. Provide a pen or pencil for each participant.
3. Challenge participants to complete the puzzle as individuals or as teams.
4. Share the correct answers as desired.

Suggestion: The puzzle may also be sent out to reinforce learning days or weeks after the lesson.

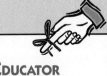

EDUCATOR SECRETS:

If you have different ability levels in your session, pair participants of opposite abilities to maximize benefits to all.

By: Kathy Harding, MSN, RN

Looking Up . . . A Child's View Crossword Puzzle

Helpful Hints for Growth and Development in Children

Across

3. A five-year-old may have magical thought processes and think illness is a _____.

5. This stage of separation anxiety can be seen in an infant who is withdrawn.

7. Anything that makes them _____ from their peers is a stressor for the adolescent.

11. The toddler, according to Erickson, strives to attain _____.

12. It is very important for the school-age child to maintain a sense of this.

14. This phase of development occurs in the infant before six months.

17. According to Erickson, the infant needs to establish this developmental task.

19. At _____ months an infant can walk with one hand held.

20. At _____ months an infant can sit steadily without support.

Down

1. This is a major stressor for children in middle infancy through preschool age.

2. The adolescent usually has the best _____ mechanism developed.

4. At _____ months an infant can walk when holding onto the furniture.

6. Infants begin to remember pain at _____ months. They associate pain with what caused it.

8. To alleviate stress for toddlers, it is important to keep their _____.

9. This fontanel usually closes by two months.

10. This stage of separation anxiety may be seen in an infant who is inconsolable.

13. The preschooler, according to Erickson, attempts to develop _____.

15. This reflex is elicited in the newborn and infancy period by stroking the cheek.

16. This fontanel is almost closed by twelve months; it is completely closed by eighteen months.

18. Infants who have reached this stage of separation anxiety may not establish trust.

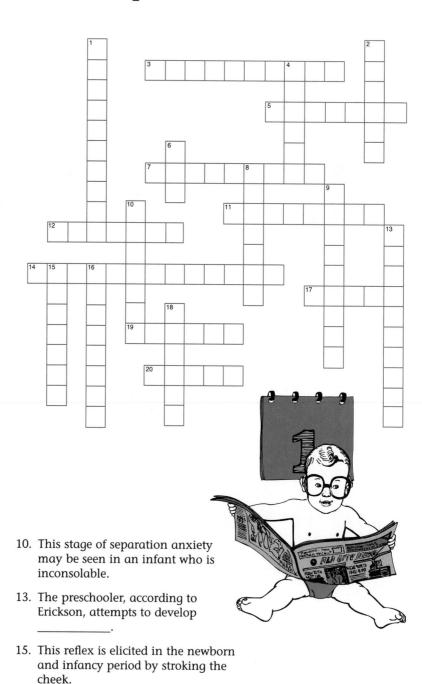

Looking Up . . . A Child's View Crossword Puzzle

Helpful Hints for Growth and Development in Children

Answer Key

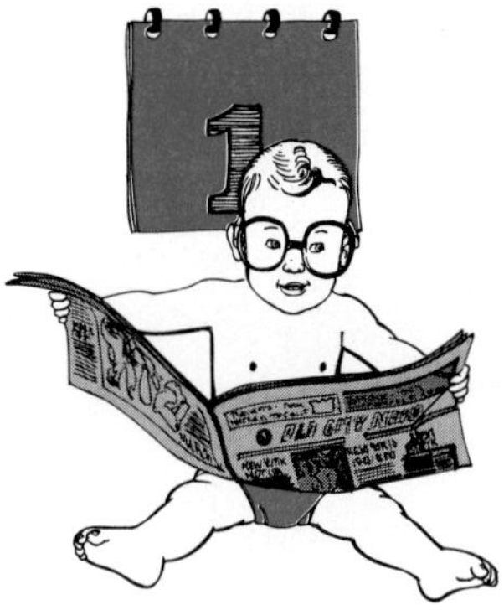

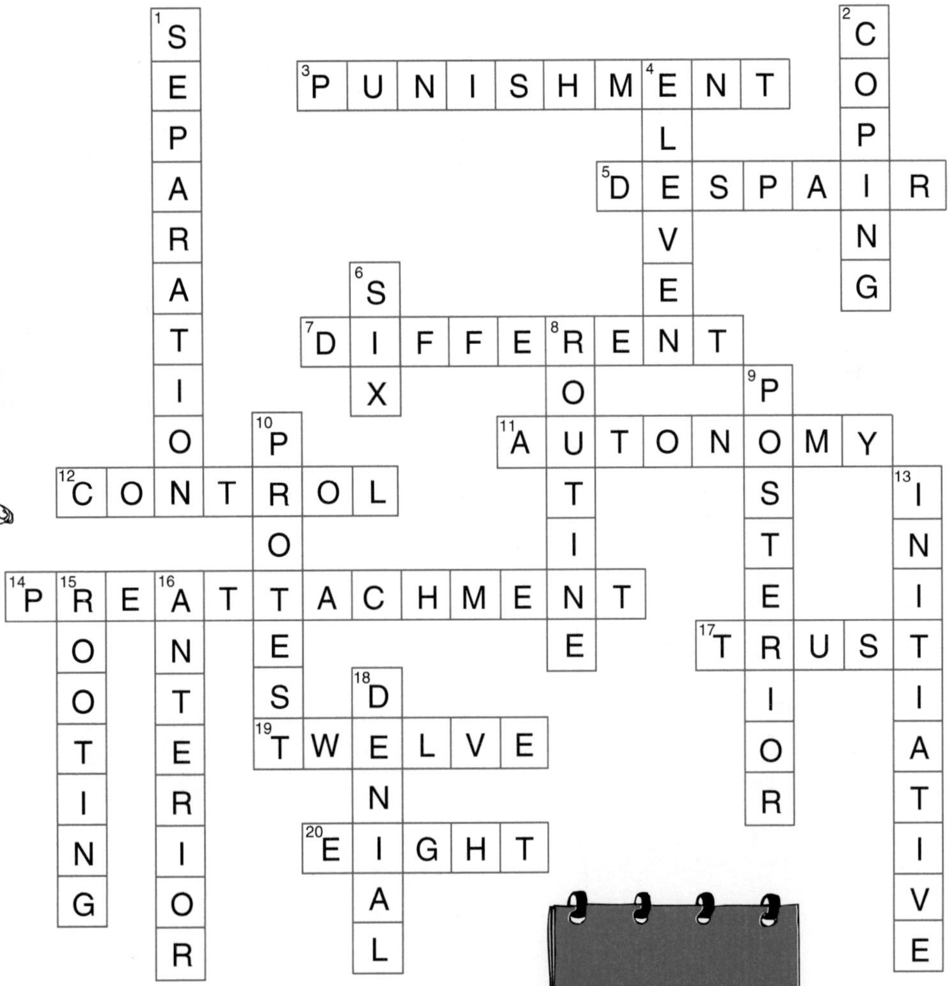

Across

3. Punishment
5. Despair
7. Different
11. Autonomy
12. Control
14. Preattachment
17. Trust
19. Twelve
20. Eight

Down

1. Separation
2. Coping
4. Eleven
6. Six
8. Routine
9. Posterior
10. Protest
13. Initiative
15. Rooting
16. Anterior
18. Denial

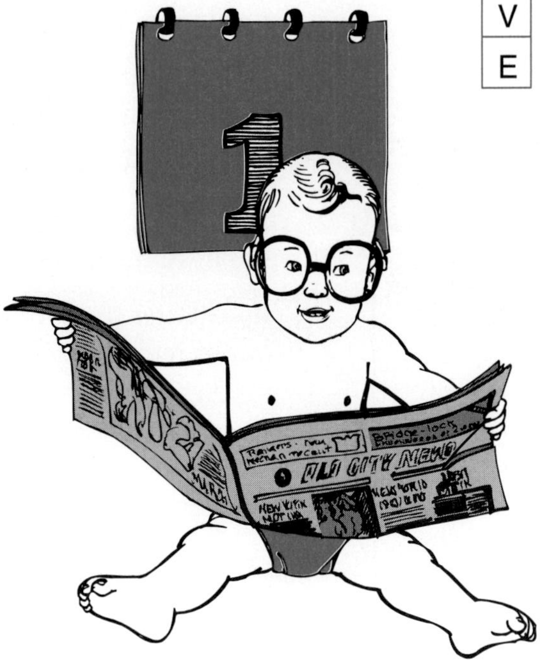

TOOL BOX

Enter The World Of Pediatrics Crossword Puzzle sheet, Enter the World of Pediatrics Crossword Puzzle Answer Key, pens or pencils

ENTER THE WORLD OF PEDIATRICS CROSSWORD PUZZLE

Preparation

1. Copy the Enter The World Of Pediatrics Crossword Puzzle for each participant.

2. Use this as an introduction to the lesson or as a review after the lesson.

3. Copy the Enter the World of Pediatrics Crossword Puzzle Answer Key.

4. Make sure all participants have a pen or pencil.

Variation: Use a poster printer copy machine to turn the crossword into a poster-size image. Plan for groups of two to six to discuss and fill in the poster-size copy of the crossword puzzle before or after your lesson.

Implementation

1. Distribute the Enter the World of Pediatrics Crossword Puzzle to each participant.

2. Provide a pen or pencil for each participant.

3. Challenge participants to complete the puzzle.

4. Share the correct answers as desired.

Hint: Enter the World of Pediatrics Crossword Puzzle may also be sent out to reinforce learning days or weeks after the lesson.

EDUCATOR SECRETS:

If you have different ability levels in your session, pair participants of opposite abilities to maximize benefits to all.

By: Kathy Harding, MSN, RN

ENTER THE WORLD OF PEDIATRICS CROSSWORD PUZZLE

Children Are Unique!

Across

3. An important nursing measure for children with respiratory disease.

5. A sign of respiratory distress. The infant or child uses accessory muscles.

6. Young infants are not able to _____ infection.

8. Infants' basal metabolic rates are _____ than the adults.

11. This portion of the airway is structurally stable due to cartilage and is called _____.

14. This is a crowing sound that indicates upper airway obstruction.

15. It is important to assess this pulse in children, especially those under two years.

16. This is often one of the first signs of hypoxia in infants and children.

Down

1. Signs of hypoxia in infants and children are very _____ initially.

2. Young infants react physiologically to stress with this type of response.

4. One gram equals how many cc's.

5. The smooth muscle of these airways constrict and dilate.

7. This is one of the first signs of hypoxia in infants and children.

9. Infants breathe via their _____ for the first four weeks of life.

10. This is a sign of respiratory distress as the infant attempts to keep the alveoli open.

12. Infants are unable to increase their respiratory depth; they _____ their rate instead.

13. Generally, the head of the bed should be _____ for clients with respiratory disease.

199

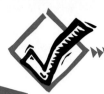

ENTER THE WORLD OF PEDIATRICS CROSSWORD PUZZLE

Children Are Unique!

Answer Key

Across

3. Positioning
5. Retractions
6. Localize
8. Faster
11. Nonreactive
14. Stridor
15. Apical
16. Tachycardia

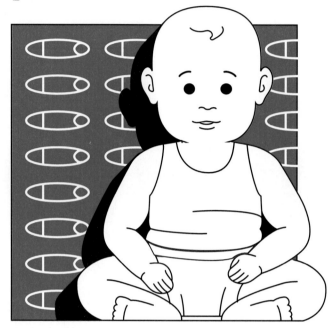

Down

1. Subtle
2. Vagal
4. One
5. Reactive
7. Tachypnea
9. Nose
10. Grunting
12. Increase
13. Elevated

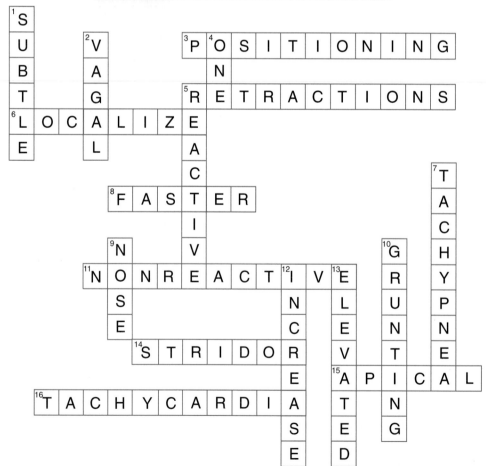

Copyright © 1998 Mosby–Year Book, Inc.

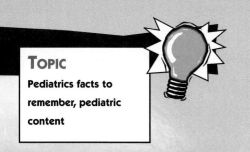

TOOL BOX
Pediatric Perils
Crossword Puzzle,
Pediatric Perils
Crossword Puzzle
Answer Key, pens
or pencils

PEDIATRIC PERILS CROSSWORD PUZZLE

Preparation

1. Copy the Pediatric Perils Crossword Puzzle for each participant.

2. Use this as an introduction to the lesson or as a review after the lesson.

3. Copy the Pediatric Perils Crossword Puzzle Answer Key.

4. Make sure all participants have a pen or pencil.

Variation: Use a poster printer copy machine to turn the crossword into a poster-size image. Plan for groups of two to six to discuss and fill in the poster-size copy of the crossword puzzle before or after your lesson.

Implementation

1. Distribute the Pediatric Perils Crossword Puzzle to each participant.

2. Provide a pen or pencil for each participant.

3. Challenge your participants to complete the puzzle.

4. Share the correct answers as desired.

Hint: Pediatric Perils Crossword Puzzle may be sent out to reinforce learning days or weeks after the lesson.

EDUCATOR
SECRETS:
If you have different
ability levels in your
session, pair
participants of
opposite abilities to
maximize benefits
to all.

By: Kathy Harding, MSN, RN

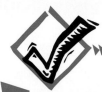

PEDIATRIC PERILS CROSSWORD PUZZLE

Facts to Remember

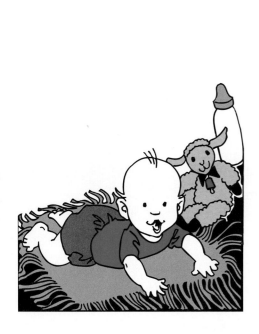

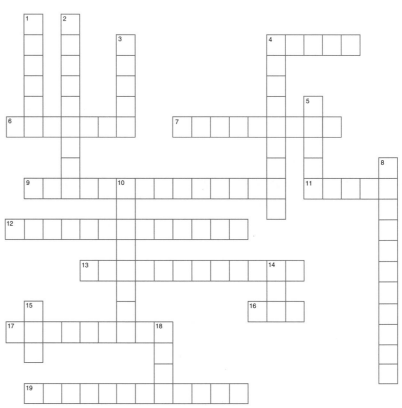

Across

4. Increases with respirations in impending respiratory distress.

6. A minor manifestation of rheumatic fever.

7. A left shift usually indicates this type of infection.

9. A genetic disease that manifests increased viscosity of exocrine glands.

11. Hold the feeding if the respirations are over _____.

12. In coarctation of the aorta, this is higher in the upper extremities than the lower ones.

13. Disease characterized by a severe sore throat and high fever.

16. An abbreviation for the condition in which the heart fails to work as a pump.

17. A child with this renal disease has proteinuria and massive edema.

19. A rise in the _____ is an indicator of impending respiratory distress.

Down

1. A prolonged expiratory phase is a symptom that is common in this disease.

2. A very common cause of gastroenteritis in children.

3. A nipple with a _____ hole may decrease fatigue during feedings for an infant with congestive heart failure.

4. A gland that aids in the digestion of food.

5. Immature neutrophils.

8. This occurs when the urethra opens along the ventral shaft of the penis.

10. A major manifestation of rheumatic fever.

14. An abbreviation for intraventricular hemorrage.

15. The lowest therapeutic level of theophylline.

18. A _____ nipple may decrease the effort expended by an infant with congestive heart failure during feeding.

PEDIATRIC PERILS CROSSWORD PUZZLE

Facts to Remember

Answer Key

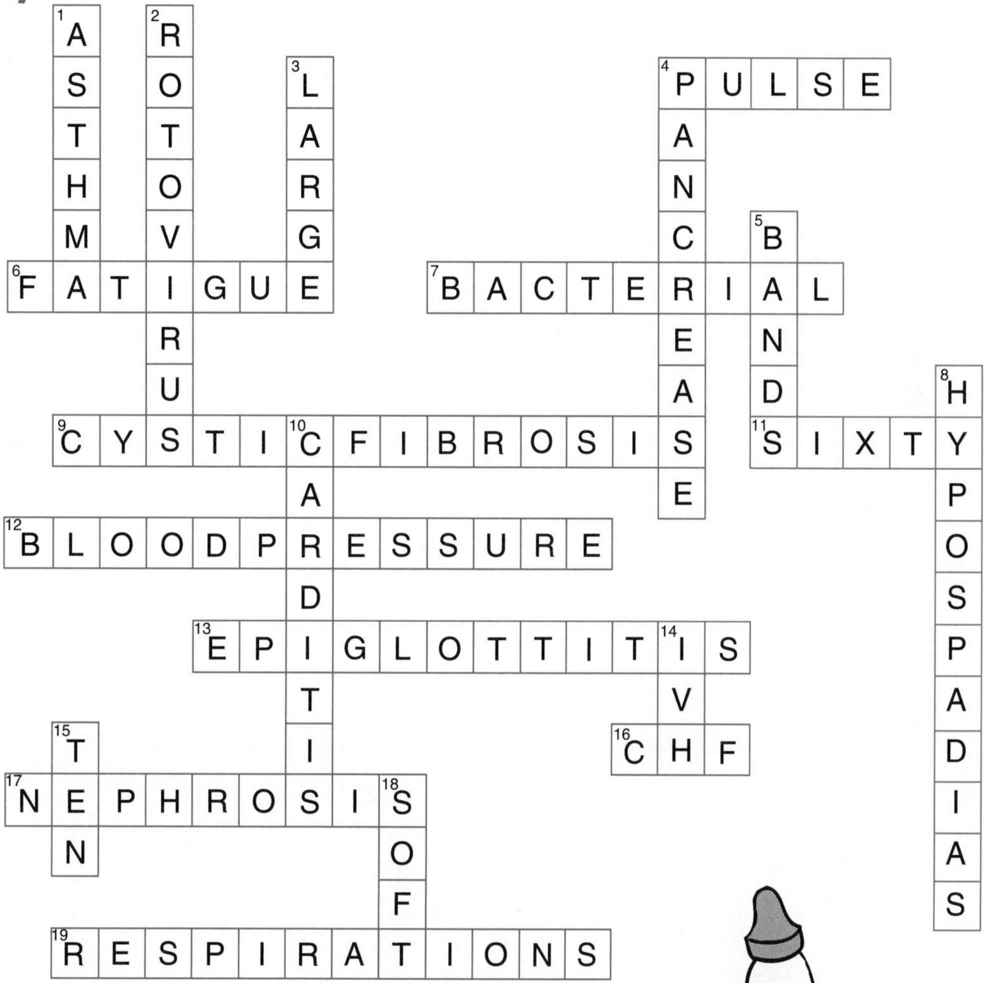

Across

4. Pulse
6. Fatigue
7. Bacterial
9. Cystic fibrosis
11. Sixty
12. Blood pressure
13. Epiglottitis
16. CHF
17. Nephrosis
19. Respirations

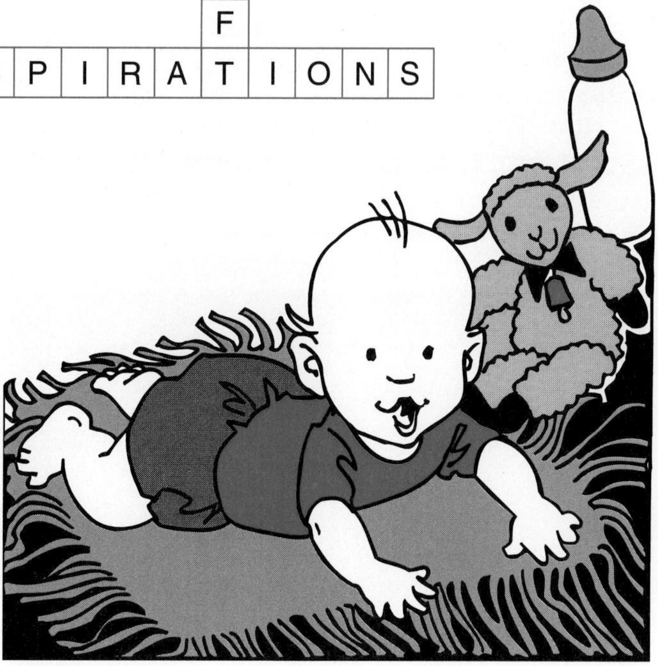

Down

1. Asthma
2. Rotavirus
3. Large
4. Pancrease
5. Bands
8. Hypospadias
10. Carditis
14. IVH
15. Ten
18. Soft

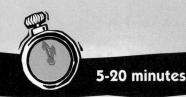

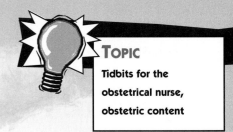

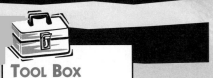

TOOL BOX

Hush Little One Crossword Puzzle, Hush Little One Crossword Puzzle Answer Key, pens or pencils

HUSH LITTLE ONE CROSSWORD PUZZLE

Preparation

1. Copy the Hush Little One Crossword Puzzle for each participant.
2. Use this as an introduction to the lesson or as a review after the lesson.
3. Copy the Hush Little One Crossword Puzzle Answer Key.
4. Make sure all participants have a pen or pencil.

Variation: Use a poster printer copy machine to turn the crossword into a poster-size image. Plan for groups of two to six to discuss and fill in the poster-size copy of the crossword puzzle before or after your lesson.

Implementation

1. Distribute the Hush Little One Crossword Puzzle to each participant.
2. Provide a pen or pencil for each participant.
3. Challenge your participants to complete the puzzle.
4. Share the correct answers as desired.

Hint: The Hush Little One Crossword Puzzle may also be sent out to reinforce learning days or weeks after the lesson.

EDUCATOR SECRETS:

If you have different ability levels in your session, pair participants of opposite abilities to maximize benefits to all.

By: Kathy Harding, MSN, RN

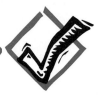

HUSH LITTLE ONE CROSSWORD PUZZLE

Tidbits for the Obstetrical Nurse

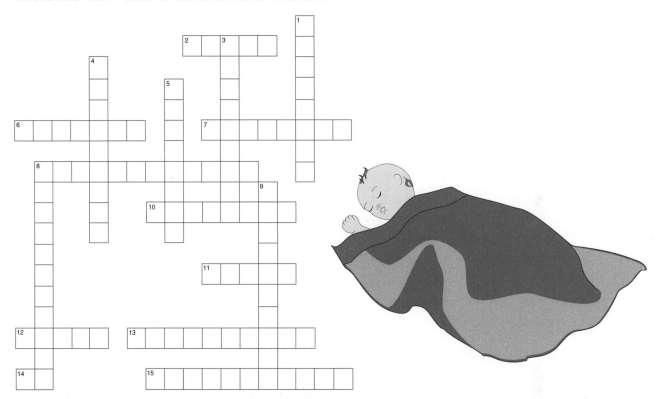

Across

2. Caused by edema of the scalp, is present at birth and may cross suture lines.

6. Noted by asymmetry of the newborn's head, resulting from the delivery process.

7. The first stool of the newborn; it is sticky, greenish black.

8. Drug given into the newborn's eyes to prevent opthalmia neonatorum.

10. This fontanel usually closes around eighteen months after birth.

11. After birth, the new mother may experience this feeling from changes in her hormones.

12. The nurse should not feed the baby if the respiratory rate is over _____.

13. Method of heat loss by contact with a cold surface.

14. Infant attachment includes the first phase, called the taking _____ phase.

15. Postpartum hemorrhage is considered when blood loss exceeds _____ cc's.

Down

1. Occurs from increased bilirubin levels resulting from the breakdown of RBCs.

3. This fontanel usually closes at nine to twelve weeks after birth.

4. Method of heat loss caused by cold surfaces not in direct contact with the body.

5. Medication given to prevent hemorrhagic disease in the newborn.

8. Method of heat loss by moisture turning into vapor.

9. Method of heat loss caused by air currents.

HUSH LITTLE ONE CROSSWORD PUZZLE

Tidbits for the Obstetrical Nurse

Answer Key

```
                                               ¹J
                        ²C A P U ³T             A
           ⁴R                    O              U
                     ⁵V          S              N
            A                    T              D
            D        I                          ⁷M E C O N I U M
⁶M O L D I N G       T           E              C
            A        A                          E
           ⁸E R Y T H R O M Y C I N
            V        I           O      ⁹C
            A        O   ¹⁰A N T E R I O R
            P        N           K      N
            O                           V
            R        ¹¹B L U E S        E
            A                           C
            T                           T
¹²S I X T Y        ¹³C O N D U C T I O N
   O                                    O
¹⁴I N              ¹⁵F I V E H U N D R E D
```

Across

2. Caput
6. Molding
7. Meconium
8. Erythromycin
10. Anterior
11. Blues
12. Sixty
13. Conduction
14. In
15. Five hundred

Down

1. Jaundice
3. Posterior
4. Radiation
5. Vitamin K
8. Evaporation
9. Convection

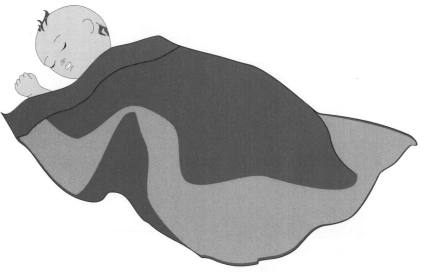

206   Copyright © 1998 Mosby–Year Book, Inc.

TOOL BOX

Postpartum Passage
Crossword Puzzle,
Postpartum Passage
Crossword Puzzle
Answer Key, pens or
pencils

POSTPARTUM PASSAGE CROSSWORD PUZZLE

Preparation

1. Copy the Postpartum Passage Crossword Puzzle for each participant.

2. Use this as an introduction to the lesson or as a review after the lesson.

3. Copy the Postpartum Passage Crossword Puzzle Answer Key.

4. Make sure all participants have a pen or pencil.

Variation: Use a poster printer copy machine to turn the crossword into a poster-size image. Plan for groups of two to six to discuss and fill in the poster-size copy of the crossword puzzle before or after your lesson.

Implementation

1. Distribute the Postpartum Passage Crossword Puzzle to each participant.

2. Provide a pen or pencil for each participant.

3. Challenge participants to complete the puzzle.

4. Share the correct answers as desired.

Hint: Postpartum Passage Crossword Puzzle may also be sent out to reinforce learning days or weeks after the lesson.

EDUCATOR SECRETS:

If you have different
ability levels in your
session, pair
participants of
opposite abilities to
maximize benefits
to all.

By: Kathy Harding, MSN, RN

POSTPARTUM PASSAGE CROSSWORD PUZZLE

Significant Facts for the Obstetrical Nurse

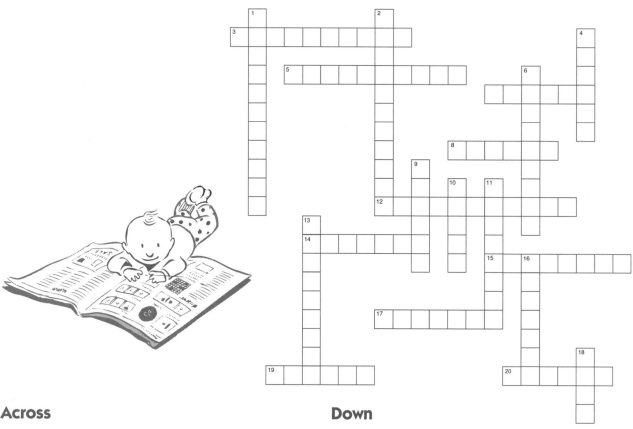

Across

3. Drug given to control bleeding in postpartum period.

5. Surgical incision into the perineum to facilitate delivery.

7. The second type of lochia, which is yellowish pink in color.

8. If criteria for administration is met, this drug must be given within 72 hours after delivery.

12. Drug used in preterm labor and can be given subq or po.

14. This vaccine should be given before or after pregnancy.

15. A drug that causes the contraction of smooth muscles.

17. Nonnarcotic analgesic used for post op pain.

19. Top portion of the uterus.

20. To properly position the infant at breast, one-half to one inch of this must be in the mouth.

Down

1. Rectal varicosities.

2. Occurs three to five days after birth, when breast tissue becomes edematous, and is a sign of lactation.

4. This sign, if positive, indicates the presence of a thrombus or thrombophlebitis.

6. Hormone responsible for milk production.

9. A patient who has a fourth-degree episiotomy may take this drug daily.

10. The first lochia, which is red in color.

11. Drug used to suppress lactation.

13. Difficulty in _____ is common after delivery, due to urethral edema.

16. Drug used in preterm labor and can be given IV or po.

18. The third type of lochia, which is white in color.

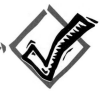

POSTPARTUM PASSAGE CROSSWORD PUZZLE

Significant Facts for the Obstetrical Nurse

Answer Key

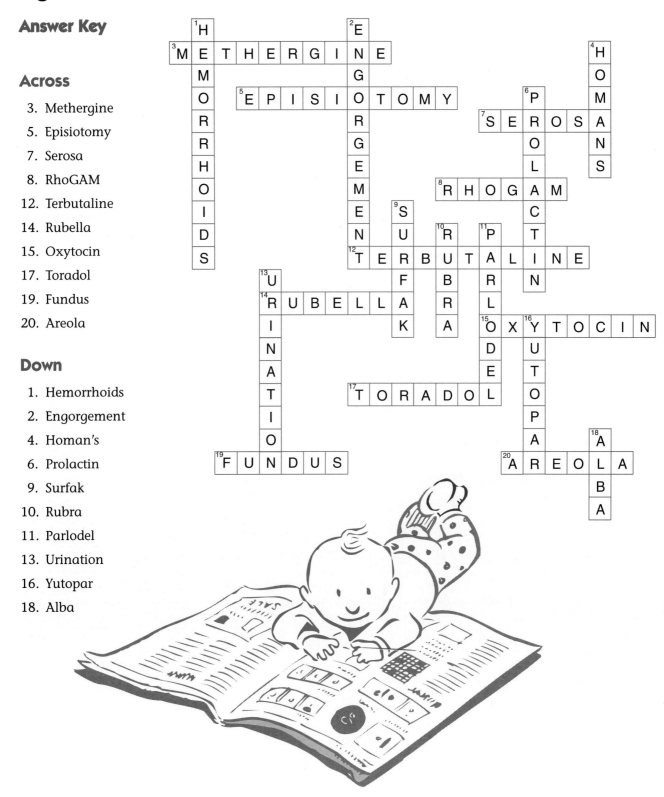

Across

3. Methergine
5. Episiotomy
7. Serosa
8. RhoGAM
12. Terbutaline
14. Rubella
15. Oxytocin
17. Toradol
19. Fundus
20. Areola

Down

1. Hemorrhoids
2. Engorgement
4. Homan's
6. Prolactin
9. Surfak
10. Rubra
11. Parlodel
13. Urination
16. Yutopar
18. Alba

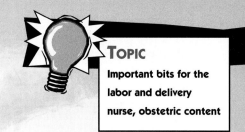

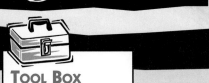

TOOL BOX

Labor and Delivery Crossword Puzzle, Labor and Delivery Crossword Puzzle Answer Key, pens or pencils

LABOR AND DELIVERY CROSSWORD PUZZLE

Preparation

1. Copy the Labor and Delivery Crossword Puzzle for each participant.

2. Use this as an introduction to the lesson or as a review after the lesson.

3. Copy the Labor and Delivery Crossword Puzzle Answer Key.

4. Make sure all participants have a pen or pencil.

Variation: Use a poster printer copy machine to turn the crossword into a poster-size image. Plan for groups of two to six to discuss and fill in the poster-size copy of the crossword puzzle before or after your lesson.

Implementation

1. Distribute the Labor and Delivery Crossword Puzzle to each participant.

2. Provide a pen or pencil for each participant.

3. Challenge your participants to complete the puzzle.

4. Share the correct answers as desired.

Hint: Labor and Delivery Crossword Puzzle may also be sent out to reinforce learning days or weeks after the lesson.

EDUCATOR SECRETS:

If you have different ability levels in your session, pair participants of opposite abilities to maximize benefits to all.

By: Kathy Harding, MSN, RN

210

LABOR AND DELIVERY CROSSWORD PUZZLE

Important Bits for the Labor and Delivery Nurse

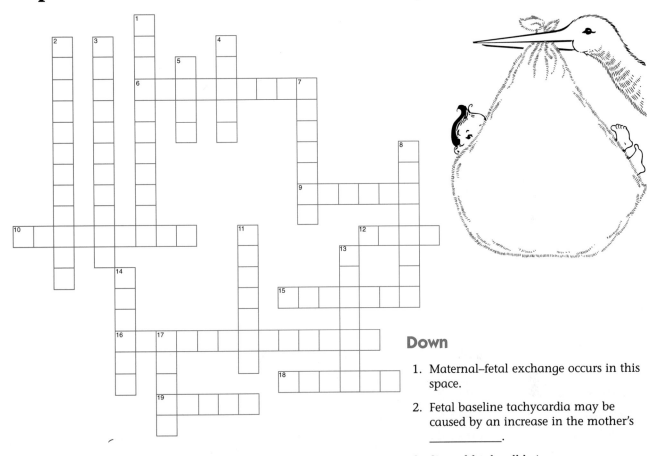

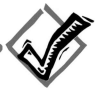

Across

6. This type of deceleration lasts 60 to 90 seconds.

9. Fetal stress may be treated with this.

10. Internal fetal monitoring can determine this type of variability.

12. Giving epidural anesthesia without hydration may cause this type of deceleration.

15. Fetal baseline tachycardia may be seen in the _____ fetus.

16. Late decelerations indicate placental _____.

18. The TOCO (can/cannot) determine the strength of a contraction.

19. This type of deceleration may indicate head compression.

Down

1. Maternal–fetal exchange occurs in this space.

2. Fetal baseline tachycardia may be caused by an increase in the mother's _____.

3. Sign of fetal well-being.

4. The influence of the vagal nerve _____ the heart.

5. Variable decelerations may be caused by compression of this.

7. The internal fetal monitor (does/does not) average fetal heart rate.

8. The external fetal monitor ultrasound transducer determines this type of variability.

11. Fetal baseline tachycardia is often the first sign of _____.

13. Drug that stimulates uterine contractions.

14. Lying a patient in the _____ position may cause late decelerations.

17. Decreased variability may be caused by a fetal _____ cycle.

LABOR AND DELIVERY CROSSWORD PUZZLE

Important Bits for the Labor and Delivery Nurse

Answer Key

Across

6. Prolonged
9. Oxygen
10. Short-term
12. Late
15. Preterm
16. Insufficiency
18. Cannot
19. Early

Down

1. Intravillus
2. Temperature
3. Variability
4. Slows
5. Cord
7. Does not
8. Long-term
11. Hypoxia
13. Pitocin
14. Supine
17. Sleep

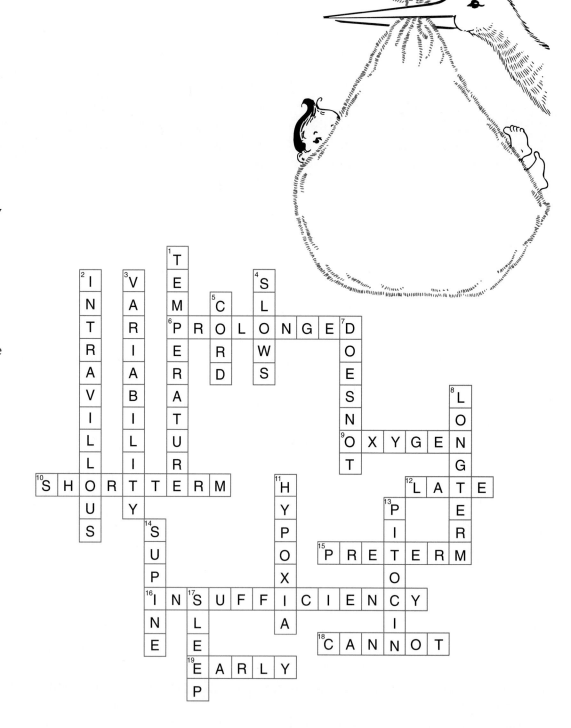

TOPIC

Teaching home health
nurses and therapists
when to involve
social workers

TOOL BOX

Transparency of the
learning facility's
specific guidelines for
involving social workers
in home care,
transparency of a social
worker referral form,
overhead projector,
pens or pencils

HOME CARE "SOCIAL"

Preparation

1. Make overhead transparencies of your facility's specific guidelines that reference when to involve social workers in home care and a social worker referral form.
2. Develop a true/false quiz based on the learning facility's or federal guidelines as to when it may or may not be appropriate to involve a social worker in a home care case.
3. Set up the overhead projector.

Implementation

1. Use the true/false quiz at the beginning of the program to create discussion about guidelines.
2. Distribute the true/false test to each participant.
3. Review and compare test results with the learning facility's and/or federal guidelines. It is interesting to discover that information everyone assumes they know may not be correct or agree with facility or federal guidelines.
4. Show and discuss the social worker referral form.

EDUCATOR SECRETS:

This idea can be used
with any guidelines and
any content.

By: Mary Arnone Cahoon, BS, RN

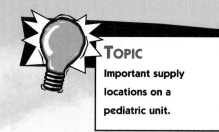

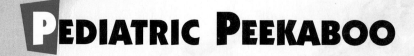

PEDIATRIC PEEKABOO

Preparation

1. Determine the number of participants or teams.

2. Make copies of Pediatric Peekaboo sheets for each participant or team.

3. Cut out boxed text from Pediatric Peekaboo sheets and make a complete set for each participant or team.

4. Store each set in an envelope.

5. Make a unit-specific location answer key after locating the following supplies:
   Pediatric drug book (PDR)
   Papoose board
   IV arm boards
   File cabinet and contents
   Blood pressure (Dynamap) machines
   Nintendo
   Nelson's *Textbook of Pediatrics*
   Scale
   Wagon
   Bandages

6. Make sure all participants have a pen or pencil.

Implementation

1. Distribute the Pediatric Peekaboo card set envelopes to each participant or team.

2. Challenge participants to solve the riddle and identify where the item can be found on their unit.

3. Ask participants to record their answers on the back of the appropriated Pediatric Peekaboo card. Participants can work individually or as teams.

4. Share the correct answers as desired.

By: Kathy Harding, MSN, RN

214

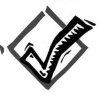

PEDIATRIC PEEKABOO

✳✳✳✳✳✳✳✳✳✳✳✳✳✳✳✳✳✳✳✳✳✳✳✳✳✳✳✳✳

I am cold to touch. I tell little ones how much they have grown each day. Who am I, and where can I be found?

✳✳✳✳✳✳✳✳✳✳✳✳✳✳✳✳✳✳✳✳✳✳✳✳✳✳✳✳✳

●●●●●●●●●●●●●●●●●●●●●●●●●●●●●●

My purpose is to inform and educate doctors and nurses. I am known as the classic pediatric text. Who am I, and where can I be found?

●●●●●●●●●●●●●●●●●●●●●●●●●●●●●●

○○○○○○○○○○○○○○○○○○○○○○○○○○○○○○

My purpose is to hug your arm real close to see what the red numbers on the machine will show. There are two sizes of me. Who am I, and where can I be found?

○○○○○○○○○○○○○○○○○○○○○○○○○○○○○○

■■■■■■■■■■■■■■■■■■■■■■■■■■■■■■

My purpose is to help little ones keep their hands and fingers from wiggling too much. Nurses put me where the special tube is and wrap me with tape or a stockinette. Who am I, and where can I be found?

■■■■■■■■■■■■■■■■■■■■■■■■■■■■■■

✺✺✺✺✺✺✺✺✺✺✺✺✺✺✺✺✺✺✺✺✺✺✺✺✺✺✺✺✺✺

My purpose is to keep little arms and legs cuddled snugly so the nurse can do procedures. Who am I, and where can I be found?

✺✺✺✺✺✺✺✺✺✺✺✺✺✺✺✺✺✺✺✺✺✺✺✺✺✺✺✺✺✺

PEDIATRIC PEEKABOO

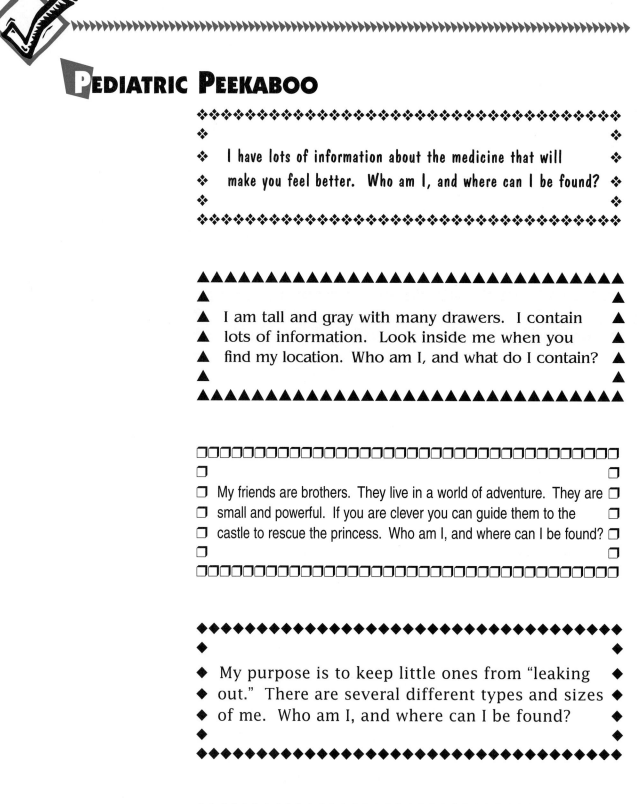

❖ I have lots of information about the medicine that will
❖ make you feel better. Who am I, and where can I be found?

▲ I am tall and gray with many drawers. I contain
▲ lots of information. Look inside me when you
▲ find my location. Who am I, and what do I contain?

❑ My friends are brothers. They live in a world of adventure. They are
❑ small and powerful. If you are clever you can guide them to the
❑ castle to rescue the princess. Who am I, and where can I be found?

◆ My purpose is to keep little ones from "leaking
◆ out." There are several different types and sizes
◆ of me. Who am I, and where can I be found?

✳ I am bright red and have four wheels. Children love
✳ me! I always need an adult with me when I'm playing.
✳ What am I, and where can I be found?

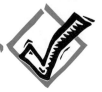

PEDIATRIC PEEKABOO

Answer Key

I am cold to touch. I tell little ones how much they have grown each day. Who am I, and where can I be found?

Scale

My purpose is to inform and educate doctors and nurses. I am known as the classic pediatric text. Who am I, and where can I be found?

Nelson's *Textbook of Pediatrics*

My purpose is to hug your arm real close to see what the red numbers on the machine will show. There are two sizes of me. Who am I, and where can I be found?

Blood pressure machine

My purpose is to help little ones keep their hands and fingers from wiggling too much. Nurses put me where the special tube is and wrap me with tape or a stockinette. Who am I, and where can I be found?

Arm board for IV

My purpose is to keep little arms and legs cuddled snugly so the nurse can do procedures. Who am I, and where can I be found?

Papoose board

217

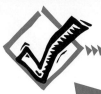

PEDIATRIC PEEKABOO

Answer Key

❖ I have lots of information about the medicine that will make you feel better. Who am I, and where can I be found?

PDR or pediatric drug book

▲ I am tall and gray with many drawers. I contain lots of information. Look inside me when you find my location. Who am I, and what do I contain?

File cabinet

❏ My friends are brothers. They live in a world of adventure. They are small and powerful. If you are clever you can guide them to the castle to rescue the princess. Who am I, and where can I be found?

Nintendo

◆ My purpose is to keep little ones from "leaking out." There are several different types and sizes of me. Who am I, and where can I be found?

Bandages

❊ I am bright red and have four wheels. Children love me! I always need an adult with me when I'm playing. What am I, and where can I be found?

Wagon

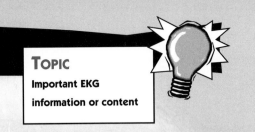
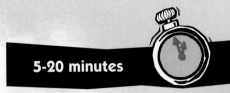

TOOL BOX
EKG Crossword Puzzle,
EKG Crossword Puzzle
Answer Key, pens
or pencils

EKG CROSSWORD PUZZLE

Preparation

1. Copy the EKG Crossword Puzzle for each participant.

2. Use this as an introduction to the lesson or as a review after the lesson.

3. Copy the EKG Crossword Puzzle Answer Key.

4. Make sure all participants have a pen or pencil.

Variation: Use a poster printer copy machine to turn the crossword into a poster-size image. Plan for groups of two to six to discuss and fill in the poster-size copy of the crossword puzzle.

Implementation

1. Distribute the EKG Crossword Puzzle sheet to each participant.

2. Provide a pen or pencil for each participant.

3. Challenge participants to complete the puzzle.

4. Share the correct answers as desired.

Hint: EKG Crossword Puzzle may also be sent out to reinforce learning days or weeks after the lesson.

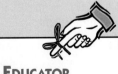

EDUCATOR
SECRETS:
If you have different
ability levels in your
session, pair
participants of
opposite abilities to
maximize benefits
to all.

By: Jeanne R. Silva, RN,
BSN, CCRN

EKG CROSSWORD PUZZLE

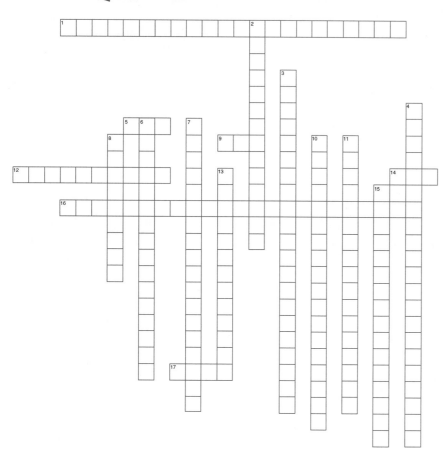

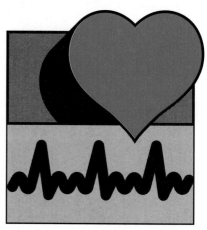

Across

1. A fast, wide complex originating from the ventricles that is often life threatening.

5. Abbreviation used to indicate an early beat from between the A-V node and the bundle of HIS.

9. Abbreviation used to indicate an early beat from the upper chambers of the heart.

12. Another name for second-degree heart block, mobitz one.

14. Abbreviation used to indicate an early beat from the lower chamber of the heart.

16. Rhythm with no identifiable complexes, just a coarse baseline that is a lethal arrhythmia.

17. Abbreviation used for wide QRS complex with no P waves and a heart rate greater than 60.

Down

2. The general term used to signify a rhythm in which the upper and lower chambers of the heart are not synchronized.

3. The name given when the P-R interval is greater than .20.

4. Wide QRS complex with no P waves and a heart rate less than 40.

6. A narrow, complex rhythm rate usually between 40 to 60 beats per minute, originating between the A-V node and the bundle of HIS.

7. An upper-chamber rhythm with no identifiable atrial wave and an irregular R-to-R interval.

8. Second-degree heart block with consistent P-R intervals and dropped beats.

10. A rhythm in which the atria is firing but is not communicating the impulses to the ventricles and the ventricle is initiating its own depolarization.

11. Rhythm between 60 to 100 beats per minute with a normal P before each QRS, and a normal and consistent PR interval.

13. Upper chamber rhythm that is regular or regularly irregular.

15. Rhythm between 100 to 160 beats per minute with a normal P before each QRS and a normal and consistent PR interval.

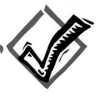

EKG CROSSWORD PUZZLE

Answer Key

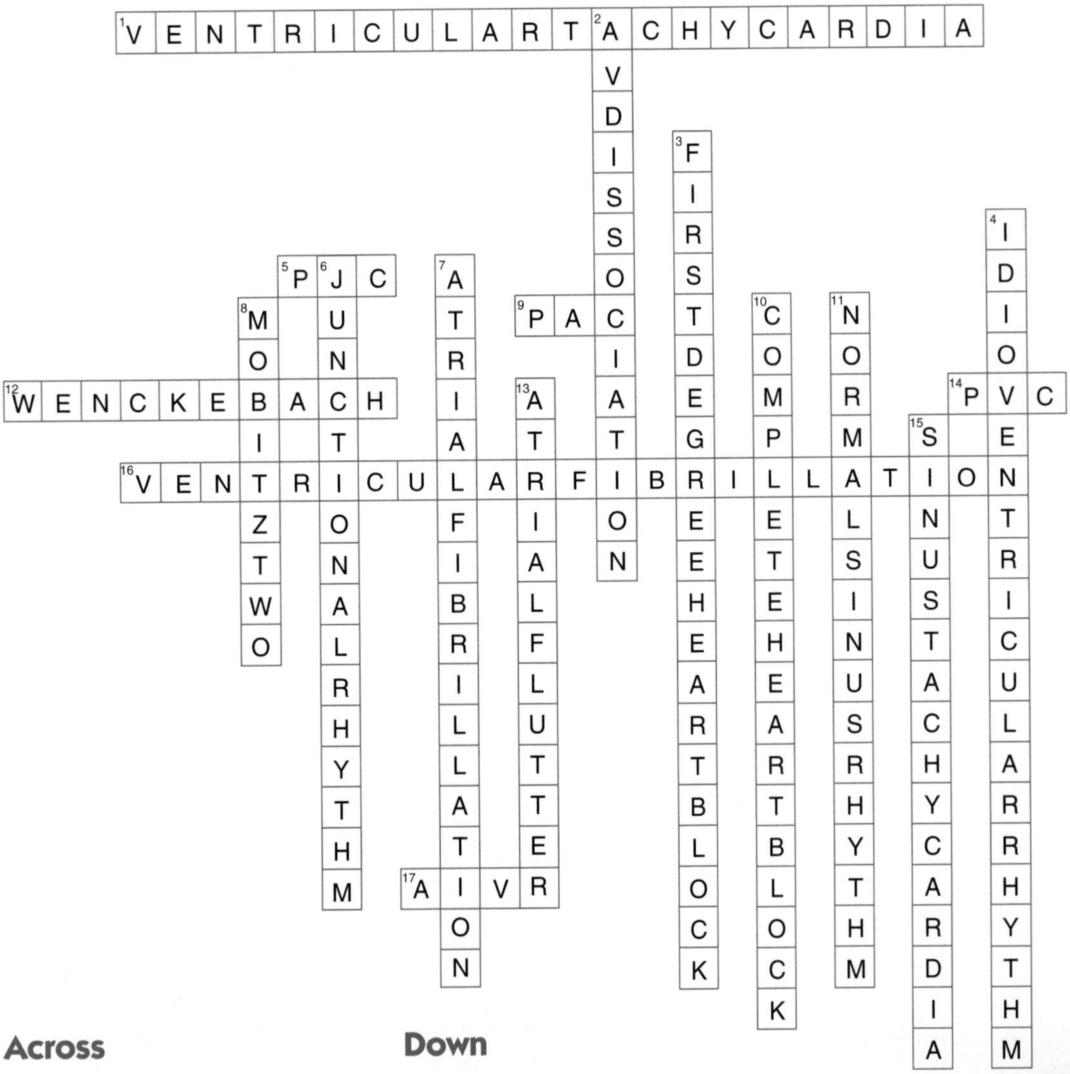

(Crossword grid — Answer Key)

Across answers: 1. VENTRICULAR TACHYCARDIA · 12. WENCKEBACH · 16. VENTRICULAR FIBRILLATION · 17. AIVR

Down answers: 2. AV DISSOCIATION · 3. FIRST DEGREE HEART BLOCK · 4. IDIOVENTRICULAR RHYTHM · 6. JUNCTIONAL RHYTHM · 7. ATRIAL FIBRILLATION · 8. MOBITZ TWO · 10. COMPLETE HEART BLOCK · 11. NORMAL SINUS RHYTHM · 13. ATRIAL FLUTTER · 15. SINUS TACHYCARDIA · 5. PJC · 9. PAC · 14. PVC

Across

1. Ventricular tachycardia
5. PJC
9. PAC
12. Wenckebach
14. PVC
16. Ventricular fibrillation
17. AIVR

Down

2. A-V dissociation
3. First-degree heart block
4. Idioventricular rhythm
6. Junctional rhythm
7. Atrial fibrillation
8. Mobitz two
10. Complete heart block
11. Normal sinus rhythm
13. Atrial flutter
15. Sinus tachycardia

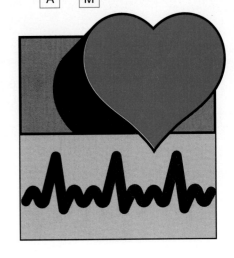

20-30 minutes

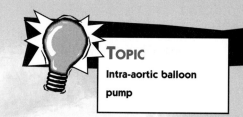

TOPIC

Intra-aortic balloon pump

TOOL BOX

IABP Questions, Not Answers Game Board, IABP Questions, Not Answers Answer Key, overhead transparency, overhead projector (or poster/flip chart), buzzing device or noisemaker, timing device, die, Post-it™ notes, small prizes or goodies

IABP QUESTIONS, NOT ANSWERS

Preparation

1. Review IABP Questions, Not Answers sheets. If the information does not agree with policies and procedures of the learning facility, edit the material to comply with that facility's policies and procedures.

2. Make an overhead transparency of the IABP Questions, Not Answers Game Board. (A poster or flip chart can be made instead, if desired.)

3. Place Post-it™ notes on all category/amount squares. This allows you to keep track of what has been chosen.

4. Make a copy of the IABP Questions, Not Answers sheet. When a team selects a category and an amount, use this sheet to read the appropriate statement.

5. Make a copy of the IABP Questions, Not Answers Answer Key. Confirm the correct answer from this sheet.

6. Obtain a buzzing device or noisemaker for each team to determine which team rings in first.

7. Obtain a timing device.

8. Collect small prizes or goodies (food such as donuts, tootsie rolls, fruit snacks, pretzels; Post-it™ notes; etc.) to award to the participants at the end of the activity.

Implementation

1. Divide the group into two or more teams of three to six participants.

2. Appoint a spokesperson or leader for each team.

3. Have the team spokesperson roll the die to determine which team will go first. (Highest number takes the lead.)

continued

EDUCATOR SECRETS:

Good to use after learning a new concept or to refresh memories.

By: Jana Magarelli, RN, MA

IABP QUESTIONS, NOT ANSWERS *continued*

4. Display the Game Board on the overhead projector. Post-it™ notes should cover all squares.

5. Explain the following rules:

   a. The spokesperson for the team selected to go first picks a category and an amount from the game board.

   b. The facilitator reads the statement from the IABP Questions, Not Answers sheet that corresponds with the selected category and amount.

   c. A team may collaborate on their response for up to five seconds. (Use the timing device to monitor this time.)

   d. The team representative states the answer in the form of a question. (See IABP Questions, Not Answers Answer Key.)

   e. If the question given is correct, the team is awarded the point(s) indicated on the IABP Questions, Not Answers Game Board.

   f. Another team may buzz in if the question is incorrect.

   g. Points are awarded for the correct question according to the amount listed on the IABP Questions, Not Answers Game Board.

6. Remove the Post-it™ notes from the category and amount squares as they are chosen.

7. Use the IABP Questions, Not Answers Answer Key to confirm the correct answer. If the answer is incorrect, you can elect to give the other team a chance to answer, or simply reveal the correct answer.

8. Award prizes to all participants.

IABP QUESTIONS, NOT ANSWERS

Game Board

Theoretical Aspects	Complications	Patient Care	Miscellaneous
1	1	1	1
2	2	2	2
3	3	3	3
4	4	4	4
5	5	5	5

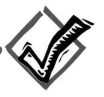

IABP QUESTIONS, NOT ANSWERS

Theoretical Aspects	Complications	Patient Care	Miscellaneous
1 The balloon assists the heart in two ways. One is to augment coronary artery perfusion and the other is this.	**1** This complication is caused by occlusion of the femoral artery, thrombus, or spasm and limits the blood flow to the distal circulation.	**1** Observation of urine output to be >30cc/hr, strict I&Os, daily BUN, creatinine, and weights. Assessment of the catheter placement on chest X-ray are all nursing intervention for this system.	**1** The most common trigger utilized is this.
2 Some contraindications to balloon pumping are irreversible brain damage and chronic end-stage heart disease. Name three others.	**2** This complication is caused by the mechanical trauma of the balloon inflation on the platelet integrity.	**2** Monitor ABG's, elevate the head of the bed 30 degrees, turning the patient, and encourage cough and deep breathing are all interventions for this system.	**2** You may need to fill the balloon more often due to elevated temperature and this.
3 Increased intracoronary blood flow, perfusion augmented to the distal circulation, and increased coronary artery perfusion indicate the balloon is properly doing this.	**3** This complication occurs when the aorta is torn during balloon insertion.	**3** Maintaining optimal diastolic augmentation and afterload reduction; rhythm strips Q2-4 hrs, vital signs Q15-30 mins, until stable; cardiac enzymes and 12-lead EKG are all interventions for this system.	**3** The wave form.
4 Reduction of the aortic end diastolic pressure, decrease in MVO$_2$, and increase in cardiac output all indicate that the balloon is properly doing this.	**4** This complication may be caused by marked hip flexion of the involved limb. A key sign when assessing is little black specks in the tubing.	**4** Peripheral pulse check Q1 hr; assessment of color and temperature of the leg involved; anticoagulation therapy; antiemboli stocking for noninvolved limb are all interventions for this system.	**4** When the "augmentation below limit" alarm sounds, the nurse's action should include this.
5 For the best results, the proper position of the balloon catheter should be here.	**5** This complication occurs after the removal of the balloon catheter. It is caused by bleeding into the surrounding tissue, resulting in constriction of that tissue.	**5** Monitor temperature Q4 hrs; observe of WBC; change insertion site dressing every day; culture of blood, urine, and insertion site for temp >101° F are all interventions for this system.	**5** During cardiac arrest the trigger of choice is this.

IABP Questions, Not Answers

Answer Key

Theoretical Aspects	Complications	Patient Care	Miscellaneous
1 What is afterload reduction?	1 What is limb ischemia?	1 What is the renal system?	1 What is the EKG trigger?
2 What are peripheral vascular disease, incompetent aortic valve, and dissecting aortic aneurysm?	2 What is thrombocytopenia?	2 What is the respiratory system?	2 What are tachyarrhythmias?
3 What is balloon inflation?	3 What is aortic dissection?	3 What is the cardiac system?	3 What is unassisted end diastole, systole, augmented diastole, assisted aortic end diastolic pressure, and assisted systole?
4 What is balloon deflation?	4 What is blood leak back in the balloon?	4 What is the vascular system?	4 What is assess the patient for decrease in cardiac output?
5 What is the descending thoracic aorta, distal to the left subclavian artery?	5 What is compartment syndrome?	5 What is the immunologic system?	5 What is pressure or internal?

HEMODYNAMIC CONCEPTS CROSSWORD PUZZLE

Preparation

1. Copy the Hemodynamic Concepts Crossword Puzzle for each participant.
2. Use this as an introduction to the lesson or as a review after the lesson.
3. Copy the Hemodynamic Concepts Crossword Puzzle Answer Key.
4. Make sure all participants have a pen or pencil.

Variation: Use a poster printer copy machine to turn the crossword into a poster-size image. Plan for groups of two to six to discuss and fill in the poster-size copy of the crossword puzzle before or after your lesson.

Implementation

1. Distribute the Hemodynamic Concepts Crossword Puzzle to each participant.
2. Provide a pen or pencil for each participant.
3. Challenge your participants to complete the puzzle.
4. Share the correct answers as desired.

Hint: Hemodynamics Concepts Crossword Puzzle may also be sent out to reinforce learning days or weeks after the lesson.

EDUCATOR SECRETS:
Great to use as homework in a critical care course.

By: Jana Magarelli, RN, MA

HEMODYNAMIC CONCEPTS CROSSWORD PUZZLE

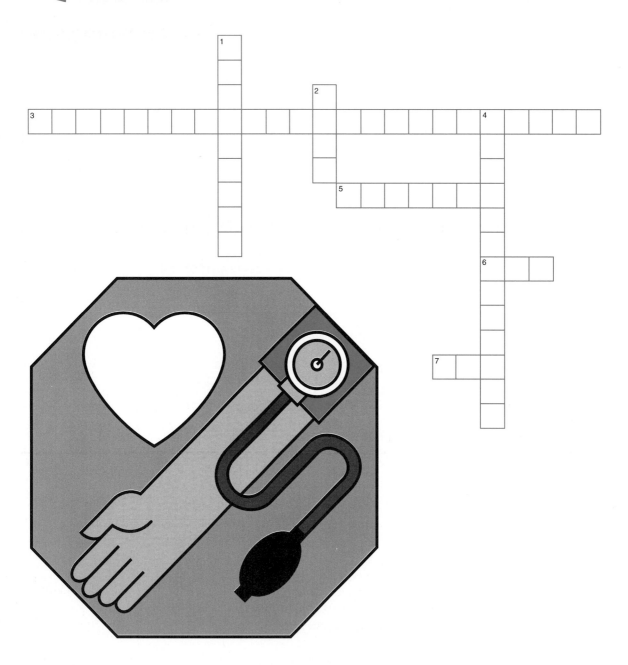

Across

3. Ventricular pressure rises without changes in volume; myocardial oxygen consumption at its highest.

5. Also known as "fiber stretch."

6. The normal values can range from 2 to 6 mmHg.

7. The normal values can range from 20 to 30 and 8 to 12 mmHg.

Down

1. Also known as "resistance."

2. The normal values range from 8 to 12 mmHg.

4. The volume of blood that is ejected from the ventricle each minute.

HEMODYNAMIC CONCEPTS CROSSWORD PUZZLE

Answer Key

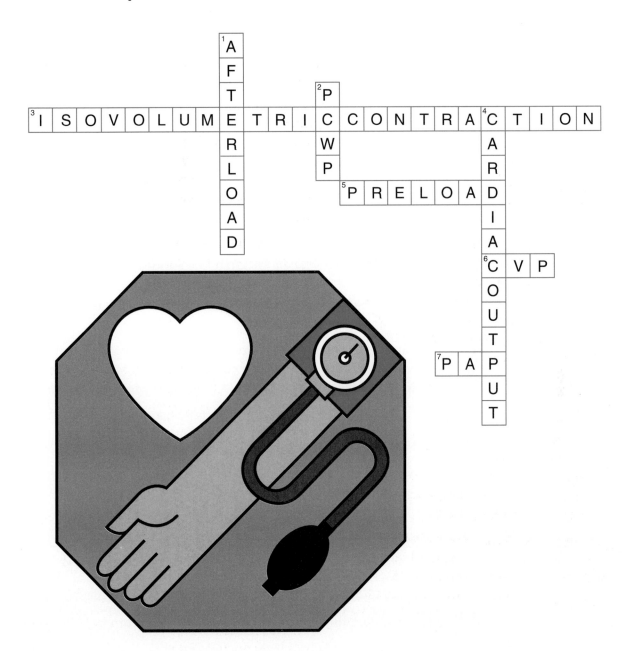

Across

3. Isovolumetric contraction
5. Preload
6. CVP
7. PAP

Down

1. Afterload
2. PCWP
4. Cardiac output

229

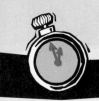

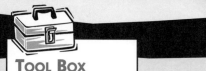

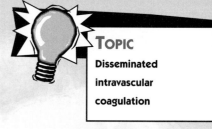

TOOL BOX

DIC Duos Numbers and Words sheets, DIC Duos Answer Key, large index cards, tape or paste, Velcro, poster board, die

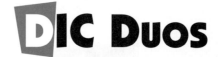

DIC DUOS

Preparation

1. Determine the number of participants and divide into two or more teams.
2. Copy DIC Duos Words sheet and cut out each box.
3. Tape or paste the words onto fourteen large, equal-sized index cards.
4. Copy DIC Duos Numbers sheet and cut out each box.
5. Tape or paste the numbers on the back of the DIC Words index cards.
6. Place a small piece of Velcro on the top middle of each card, front and back.
7. Place pieces of Velcro throughout the poster board so the index cards can be attached in numerical order.

Variation: Place a picture or rebus puzzle on the poster board so that participants have something to solve at the end of the round. Make sure the picture or puzzle is difficult to solve so that all matches are made before the puzzle is solved.

Implementation

1. Divide the group into two or more teams.
2. Have each team choose a spokesperson.
3. Allow the spokesperson for each team to roll a die to determine which team goes first.
4. Ask the lead team's spokesperson to call out a number from one to fourteen.
5. Turn over the called number card, read it, and show it to participants.
6. Ask the same team to find the match for the revealed card by calling out a second number.
7. Turn over the card, read it, and show it to participants. If the cards match, the picking team must explain why they match to gain a point. Both the match and the explanation must be achieved to maintain playing status. If the match and the explanation are not complete, play moves to the other team.
8. Continue play until all the matches are complete and the board is clear.

EDUCATOR SECRETS:

Great review after class. Laminate the cards for reuse.

By: Jana Magerilli, RN, MA

230

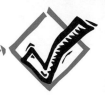

DIC Duos

Numbers

1	2
3	4
5	6
7	8
9	10
11	12
13	14

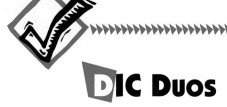

DIC Duos

Words

Factor VIII	Antihemophilic factor
Factor IV	Diagnosis
Extrinsic pathway	Platelets
Calcium	Three or more unrelated areas of bleeding and abnormal lab values
Hypertensive, shocky, and bleeding	150,000 to 400,000 mm³
1:4 or <10	Hypertensive, shocky, and bleeding
Fibrin split product	Presentation

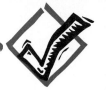

DIC Duos

Factor VIII	Antihemophilic factor
Factor IV	Calcium
Extrinsic pathway	Activated by injury to tissue and vessel
Diagnosis	Three or more unrelated areas of bleeding and abnormal lab values
Platelets	150,000 to 400,000 mm^3
Presentation	Hypertensive, shocky, and bleeding
Fibrin split product	1:4 or <10

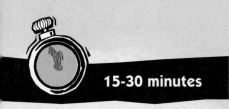

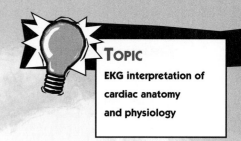

15-30 minutes

TOOL BOX

Notes on story using "kingdom" descriptors

THE KING AND QUEEN OF HEARTS

Preparation

1. Review cardiac anatomy and physiology associated with EKG rhythms before a teaching session.

2. Practice using the "kingdom" descriptors (see *Implementation*) before class so that you are comfortable with them.

Implementation

Explain the origin of sinus, atrial, junctional, and ventricular beats as they relate to cardiac anatomy by telling a story using "kingdom" descriptors.

1. The sinus node is king, a constant ruler, in charge until death, until . . .

2. The atria, or queen, takes over. This only happens if the king becomes weak or distracted.

3. If the king and the queen are both weak or distracted, the wicked sorcerer takes over as junctional beats.

4. If the queen becomes upset with the king, she'll let him know it by a premature atrial contraction.

5. The subjects of the kingdom grow restless occasionally and let the king know by throwing stones, or premature ventricular contractions. This can be harmless, until . . .

6. Several subjects become disenchanted and take over as ventricular tachycardia, which can further develop into . . .

7. Chaos, as subjects fight even among themselves, or ventricular fibrillation.

8. If the sorcerer has a planned effort to slow down the activity of the king, a first-degree A-V block occurs.

9. If the king and sorcerer are having problems communicating, a second-degree heart block occurs.

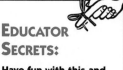

EDUCATOR SECRETS:

Have fun with this and refer to it when a participant is having difficulty with these concepts.

continued

By: Julia Aucoin, MN, RN, C

THE KING AND QUEEN OF HEARTS   *continued*

10. Anarchy develops between the king and kingdom and they function independently as a third degree complete heart block.

11. If the king has remained in power and dies a natural death, he will wave good bye to his subjects through an agonal rhythm.

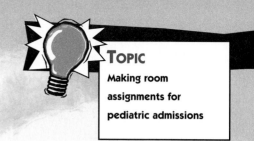

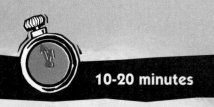

TOOL BOX

Admission Shuffle
Pediatric Floor Map,
Admission Shuffle
Pediatric Patient Tokens

THE ADMISSION SHUFFLE

Preparation

1. Copy the Admission Shuffle Pediatric Floor Map.
2. Make copies of the Admission Shuffle Pediatric Patient Tokens.
3. Cut out the Admission Shuffle Pediatric Patient Tokens squares.
4. Make extra Admission Shuffle Pediatric Patient Tokens, if desired, using the blank squares.

Implementation

1. Review the factors that are important when making room assignments for pediatric patients: age, sex, and diagnosis (isolation, need for observation).
2. Place the Admission Shuffle Pediatric Patient Tokens face down in a pile.
3. Place the Admission Shuffle Pediatric Floor Map in the middle of the group, and point out the four semiprivate and two private rooms.
4. Begin the game by modeling for the participants: Take a card, assign a room, and state your reason for the specific room assignment to the group.
5. Have each participant take a turn drawing a Pediatric Patient Token from the token pile and have them assign the room, place the token on the floor map, and state their reason.
6. Allow other participants or yourself to assist with an explanation if a participant is unfamiliar with the diagnosis.
7. Discuss the room assignment as a group and allow participants to change room assignments as a result of the discussion.
8. Notice when the floor fills up. Initiate a discussion on what options are available at the participants' facility. As the facilitator, you may occasionally discharge patients by removing tokens from the Admission Shuffle Pediatric Floor Map.

Suggestion: The game's complexity can be increased by discussing staffing needs with each addition.

continued

EDUCATOR SECRETS:

This game works well as a clinical conference activity.

By: Terry Delpier, MN, RN, CPNP

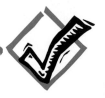

THE ADMISSION SHUFFLE

Pediatric Floor Map

Nurse Station		Room 1
		Room 2
Room 5 (Private)		Room 3
Room 6 (Private)		Room 4

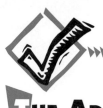

THE ADMISSION SHUFFLE

Pediatric Patient Tokens

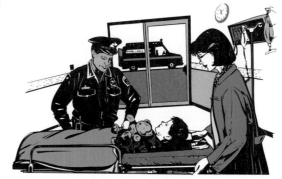

2 months female FTT	2 years female r/o meningitis	4 years male VSD, Down's r/o endocarditis	18 months male gastro dehydration
4 years female asthma	6 months female r/o sepsis HIV+	2 months male developmental dysplasia of the hip Bryant's tx	6 years male all on chemo ANC <500
3 years female VSD post cath	4 months female bronchiolitis	2 months male bronchiolitis	16 years male post op appy
13 years female migraines neuro workup dark, quiet room ordered	6 years female post op T&A 6-hour stay requested private	14 years male post op arthroscopy	10 years male fractured femur in skeletal tx

THE ADMISSION SHUFFLE

Pediatric Patient Tokens

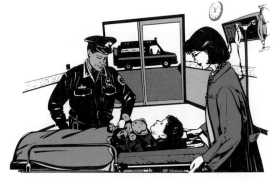
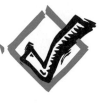

7 years female diabetes new dx	11 years female spina bifida post op VP shunt revision	2 months male post op cleft lip repair	2 years male MRI sedation r/o brain tumor
16 years female post MVA GT, trach	9 years female CF cleanout	5 years male sickle cell crisis	1 year male r/o Wilms' tumor
8 years female post op tendon release CP, GT	7 months female croup	3 years male seizures unknown origin	7 years male osteomyelitis
2 months female r/o GER apnea	3 years female post op ureter re-implantation	2 years male r/o Kawasaki disease	4 years male nephrotic syndrome

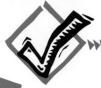

THE ADMISSION SHUFFLE

Pediatric Patient Tokens

Directions: Create your own patient scenarios.

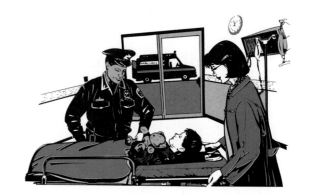

TOPIC

Values, values
clarification,
appreciation of other's
values, recognizing and
accepting ambivalence

TOOL BOX

Where Do I Stand
Questions/Scenarios;
"Yes," "No," and
"Undecided" signs
(optional)

WHERE DO I STAND?

Preparation

1. Copy the Where Do I Stand? signs.

2. Examine your room setting to ensure easy mobility from one area of the room to another (such as electrical cords, tables, etc.).

3. Hang the signs in three areas of the room.

4. Copy the Where Do I Stand? Questions/Scenarios to Consider for your use.

5. Select the questions/scenarios you plan to use.

Implementation

1. Identify the designated "Yes," "No," and "Undecided" areas of the room to your participants.

2. Instruct participants that you will read a statement and they will respond by going to the area of the room that corresponds to their belief.

3. Read each statement, allowing time in between for participants to move to their chosen area.

EDUCATOR SECRETS:

Allowing participants to offer comments or questions during the activity can enhance the learning. This will add time and must be considered when planning the learning session.

By: Jeri L. Ashley, RN,
MSN, AOCN

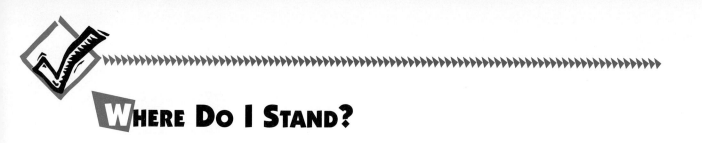
Yes

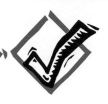
No

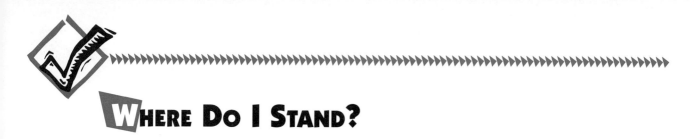

Undecided

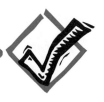

WHERE DO I STAND?

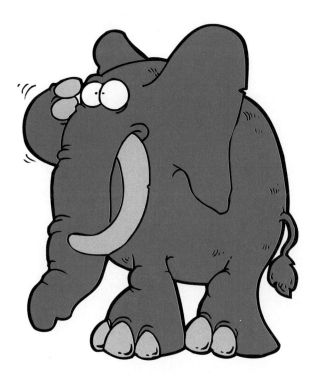

Questions/Scenarios to Consider

1. If I were out of work and unable to find a job, I would take a job with a large weapons maker.

2. You have been offered a large sum of money to be a surrogate mother, and you need the money. Would you do it?

3. I fully support interracial marriages.

4. A baby is born with incurable disorders and is in extreme pain. Would you be involved in prescribing or administering an overdose?

5. The family of a patient with a terminal illness begs you to keep it from the patient. When the patient asks you, do you tell the truth?

6. You suspect your neighbor is abusing her children. Do you notify authorities?

7. A waitress in a restaurant forgets to add $6.00 in drinks to your bill. Do you remind her?

8. You discover a medication error made by a peer where no damage occurred. Do you report it?

9. I believe that terminally ill patients have the right to take their own life.

10. I believe that patients should always be told the truth about their cancer and their prognosis.

11. I believe that nutrition should be withheld at the terminal patient's request.

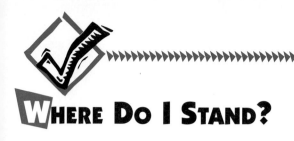

WHERE DO I STAND?

Questions/Scenarios to Consider

12. I believe the nurse should be a patient advocate at all times.

13. Families that withhold information from their loved ones need to be supported.

14. Nurses should be emotionally involved with their patients.

15. It is acceptable for a nurse to become romantically or sexually involved with a patient.

16. Adult children have the right to withhold medical treatment from their elderly parents.

17. Parents have the right to withhold medical treatment from their young children.

18. I believe in fetal organ donation.

19. I believe in capital punishment.

20. I believe teens who commit violent crimes should consistently be tried as adults in a court of law.

21. You suspect a nursing assistant of making up vital signs on a very difficult and demanding patient. Do you report the assistant?

22. The cashier in the hospital cafeteria gives you back 50 cents more that you deserve. Do you give it back?

23. An African-American child has been living happily with a white family for three years. Now the natural relatives want to take the child back. Do you believe the child should go to the birth parents?

24. A white child has been living happily with an African-American family for three years. Now the natural relatives want to take the child back. Do you believe the child should go to the birth parents?

25. I believe that a patient's confidentiality should be maintained at all costs, regardless of harm to others.

26. You work 11 to 7 on a hospital unit. You discover a patient's diary, and the patient is sound asleep. Do you read it?

27. A nurse working on your unit frequently has an offensive body odor. Do you tell the nurse?

28. You know you are attractive. Do you use sex to get ahead in your career?

29. You are an unmarried woman who desperately wants a child. Would you try to get pregnant by a one-time lover without getting his consent?

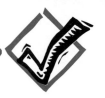

Where Do I Stand?

Questions/Scenarios to Consider

30. Would you encourage your 16-year-old unmarried daughter to have an abortion?

31. On a cold winter day, you notice a bum who has passed out on a sidewalk. Do you try to help him?

32. Would you change your religion in order to marry someone you love?

33. The neighbor next door to your apartment is beating his wife. Do you call the police?

34. Could you shoot and kill someone who has broken into your house and is threatening harm to you or your family?

35. A friend asks you to write a letter of reference for a job you feel he is poorly qualified to do. Do you write the letter?

36. Your child tells you that he or she is gay. Do you try to talk your child out of it?

37. Your spouse has been unfaithful. Do you leave the relationship?

38. You are running errands. You have one left to do before arriving for an important appointment, and you are running out of time. The only available parking spot is reserved for the handicapped. Do you park there?

39. You are involved in a car accident resulting in a few bruises, but no other injuries. Your lawyer tells you that you can get a much larger settlement if you exaggerate your injuries. Do you do this?

40. You are caring for a terminally ill patient who is experiencing a great deal of pain. The doctor prescribes a large dose of morphine, which could take the patient's life. Do you give it?

41. You have a sexual fling while on an out-of-town business trip. Do you tell your spouse?

42. The husband of a critically ill elderly woman who is ventilator dependent offers you $10,000 to assist in ending his beloved wife's life. Do you accept? Do you report this?

43. A patient tearfully reports to you that her doctor made sexual advances toward her. The physician is well respected in the community as a doctor and as a deacon in the local Episcopal church. Do you report it?

44. A nurse has a severe case of bad breath. Do you tell the nurse?

45. A doctor has a severe case of bad breath. Do you tell the doctor?

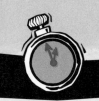

15 minutes

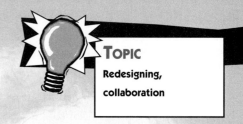

TOOL BOX

Strategies for Enhancing
Collaboration, Two
Strategies for Enhancing
Collaboration
worksheet, envelopes

COLLABORATION IDEAS

Preparation

1. Review Strategies for Enhancing Collaboration. Make revisions if statements do not agree with the learning facility's guidelines.

2. Determine the number of teams (four to six participants per team).

3. Copy Strategies for Enhancing Collaboration for each team.

4. Cut each strategy for collaboration into single strips (a set contains all strategies).

5. Place each set in an envelope.

6. Copy the Two Strategies for Enhancing Collaboration worksheet for each participant.

Implementation

1. Divide participants into small teams of four to six participants.

2. Recruit or appoint a team leader.

3. Distribute one envelope per team.

4. Inform participants that each envelope contains ideas to enhance interdepartmental collaboration.

5. Ask each person to silently read each idea, passing the ideas around their team until everyone has read all of the ideas.

6. Distribute the Two Strategies for Enhancing Collaboration worksheet.

7. Instruct participants to select what they think are the two best ideas, and record their ideas on the Two Strategies for Enhancing Collaboration worksheet.

8. Debrief the ideas with the group.

**EDUCATOR
SECRETS:**

Consider offering a
reward to the first three
people who implement
their ideas and call or
write to you about their
results.

By: Pamela Brown Stewart,
MN, RN, CCRN

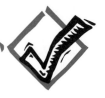

STRATEGIES FOR ENHANCING COLLABORATION

Identify someone in your organization that you don't know very well that has duties and responsibilities similar to yours. Invite that person to lunch to discuss ways you could work together.

Attend an education committee meeting for a department other than your own. Look for activities that could be expanded to other parts of the organization.

Invite staff from another service or department to an in-service that would be relevant to their care or service area, such as inviting the admissions office staff to the ICU in-service on advanced directives.

Invite staff from several different departments to serve as presenters at in-services and continuing education programs.

Co-sponsor an in-service or continuing education program with other departments. This gives both planners and participants a chance to collaborate.

Invite educators and department leaders to an open house to view the current program being used for clinical staff competency assessment and validation.

Organize an organization-wide investigation and inventory of tools and resources available for assessing, evaluating, maintaining, improving, and documenting staff competency.

Two Strategies for Enhancing Collaboration

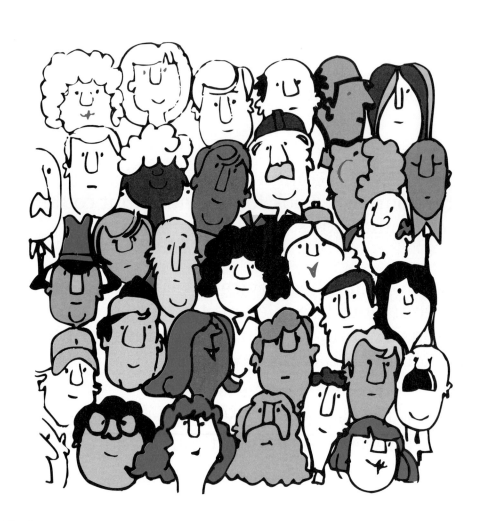

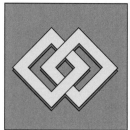

_____

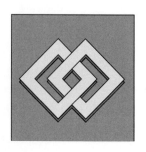

_____

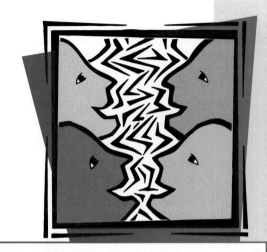

PART 5

ADVICE FROM EXPERIENCE

ADVICE FROM EXPERIENCE

So you've read this book and now face an important decision. Where do you start? The best advice I can offer from experience is to first pick an idea that you like and would enjoy doing. Look at the current content areas you are called on to deliver and ask, "What part is not working or is ineffective in getting the message across? What part of the information is so boring, dry, or complex, even I can't stand to hear it again?" Choose this one block of content for use with an instant teaching tool. You'll notice that you will look forward to teaching with that idea as a breath of fresh air to you and your participants. Since you are beginning with a part of the content that needs some help, you have nothing to lose and everything to gain!

The next step I would suggest is to increase your comfort level with the tool before you use it if you've never used an interactive exercise before. Practice administering it to your family, friends, or work colleagues so that you can get the explanation clear and all the bugs worked out. This will increase your comfort level with the tool. You might visualize, or give yourself a short mental rehearsal, of what happens first, second, and so on. Your familiarity and attitude of success is a crucial component in the process. It is an important key to success in any area of life.

After this initial educator hurdle, it will become very easy to quickly insert an instant teaching tool into an educational offering. Each of the instant tools list the items needed, as well as the preparation and implementation steps. It will not take the same amount of time and confidence investment the very first one does. Use a new teaching tool each time you perform an old program. You'll be amazed at the results.

Many people ask me how to best utilize these tools with serious, academic, or left-brained audiences who don't like anything that is called a game. There are three things I employ when facing these groups of learners. The first thing I do is to start at their comfort level with content delivery. That means if they are used to the traditional methods of slides and lecture only, I will deliver the first seven to twenty minutes in that mode. Once they are comfortable with me, then I will quote statistics for them, which I consider step two in the process. "In a moment, we will experience a high-retention, adult learning methodology that will increase your retention of content up to ninety percent in thirty days." This makes sense to them. The third thing I do is a low-risk activity that they can engage in as a small group team member, not as a lone individual. By low risk, I mean something that resembles an adult-type activity, such as a crossword puzzle, game show–type activity or a thinking puzzle. The reason I ask them to do the activity with a partner or small group is so that a positive human bond or connection is made and the learning risk is lowered. The contributions of more than one person makes that possible.

One of the many secrets I know about teaching adults involved in health care is that I never refer to any of these activities as a *game*. I've even taken to calling it the *"g" word.* I substitute many different and acceptable terms for it, such as: receipt-of-information project, reinforcing activity, energizing content delivery, and so forth. The reason for this is because there are some learners out there who do not know that a game can easily teach them something in a very enjoyable way. They think learning must be painful, boring, and a hardship to endure. Somewhere in their past they came to believe that a game was a waste of time rather than a very productive learning vehicle. People seem to have an emotional response to the word *game*. Some think it means that there is a chance they will lose at something. From the descriptions of the instant teaching tools here, everyone wins because everyone learns. That's the educator's bottom line. I've eliminated that emotional response by not speaking the *"g"* word in a teaching capacity.

What are some of the results you'll see when incorporating instant teaching tools? Learners will comment on how nice it was to enjoy a learning experience. They will compliment you on how well the lesson went. Your evaluations will show a trend to a higher average score. The "old timers" who return to mandatory education will speak in appreciative tones that you have found a fun way to present the same old information. Learners even remark on how quickly the time passed in comparison to other offerings they have attended. There will occasionally be someone who does not like your new style and will tell you so. That's okay. It is impossible to please all of the people all of the time, but it is best to please the greater majority. I'm sometimes amazed at educators' reactions to the evaluation of programs, anyway. They can quote the one or two negative remarks people wrote about them five years ago, but rarely can they quote any, much less all, of the positive ones. I have a personal policy on how I handle class or sessions evaluations now after seventeen years of teaching. I do not read them until the next day, no matter what. I never glance at them when learners are around because I am so easy to read. It is hard for me to hide my disappointment when I tell them goodbye if I know they have given me a particularly poor evaluation. When collecting evaluations, I don't even glance at the forms, but I store them in an envelope overnight. I ask myself some important, yet hard questions. Did I try my best? Did I adequately prepare? Is my sense that most participants had a positive experience? Did any part of the class make me cringe? What can I improve next time? Once answering these honestly for myself, the next day I read each evaluation and take to heart all advice offered. Some of the best growth opportunities present themselves in the words of our participants. Even negative evaluations can be vehicles to take us to the next level of performance. If a comment is said by two or more, I really try to focus on improving that area.

Another benefit of using these instant teaching tools is the difference it will make to you, the educator. It will challenge you to broaden your experience in the use of a variety of teaching methods. It will reawaken the desire to teach effectively and to see positive evidence of it occurring. It can be tracked and measured, with better overall retention results over lecture-based teaching. You can begin to see more clearly that what you do when you educate is that you make a difference. Your impact increases and that challenges you to do even more projects in an effective way. It is possible to develop and appreciate a love of life-long learning, which is the future for all of us.

What do you do if the tool you've chosen isn't the right one for the information or group, and you're in the middle of it. Don't be afraid to shift gears in the middle. Rarely have I seen this actually happen, but some educators express this fear. Feel free to smile, stay positive, and move on!

Part of the reason I think this happens so rarely in my experience is because I really believe these work! I've seen it hundreds of times with many diverse groups. I think learners can sense when you are unsure and nervous, and it invites them (if they are a group of sharks) to attack. I pretend in my head and act as if there is no chance for a negative outcome, and they sense that confidence and respond to it. I do not apologize for any reason, and I maintain positive words about any outcome or response I receive. I remember asking a group of educators to brainstorm a list of benefits to using these types of teaching tools. One person stood up and said the opposite, with the words, "It will take too much time!" How should you respond? This is what I said, "Jane, you have raised an excellent point, that is, always be aware of selecting short time-frame activities when under time constraints." I chose to see the positive side of that comment and later shared four ways to gain time when teaching a large quantity of content with time constraints because I then knew it was a concern. It actually can take people less time to learn information through an activity than traditional methods. How is that possible? People have a higher retention rate when learning in an activity than just hearing it said once. Information just said to a group must go through multiple repetitions to actually be retained. All it takes is planning time, not actual delivery time, to use an instant teaching tool.

It is sometimes best to set your learners up in teams for these activities. Exactly how many people do you need to make a team? It can be a team of just two or multiple teams of up to six members.

This creates a safety zone in which to take a learning risk. Everyone can be involved simultaneously, so that no one feels left out or embarrassed. It allows the members to tap into the skills and knowledge of each member, no matter how diverse. I use the strategy of mixing up the members of each team so that they are not on a team with their friends or workmates, but with members of different departments, cultural backgrounds, and knowledge and experience levels. This levels the playing field for all so that they can hear a variety of challenges and information throughout the session. A new knowledge and level of appreciation can be shared between units or areas that have faced conflict in the past. An equalization of personal dynamics occurs. Everyone must meet new people; no one group has a history or advantage over another. This secretly breaks up groups of negative people who find safety in numbers and can be negative in a group of supporters. If they are divided, it is harder to be the lone voice of negativity in a crowd. This is an educator secret, never to be told to learners. We can orchestrate the dynamics so that everyone has the best possible learning experience, not just those who come and stay with their friends.

One other tool for success of these activities is to begin by teaching a refocus signal to your participants. This will allow you to quickly refocus their attention when time for an activity is up without straining your voice or wasting time. What is a refocus signal? It can be a bell, whistle, chime, clap, or physical sign such as a hand raised in the air. This way, when you need their attention there is no confusion or time wasted in obtaining it.

I challenge you to take a risk. Try some new and different tools. You may have a history of using creative ideas such as these. In that case, try some of the ones you find more challenging to use. Why? If you never take a learning risk, you cannot grow. Our ultimate goal is to improve the knowledge and skill of others as well as ourselves. We often ask others to change their knowledge, skills, and attitudes. How can we truly appreciate how hard a task that is if we can't or won't do it ourselves? The key to being an outstanding educator is to stay a learner. The more we grow comfortable and bored with our teaching, the less effective our message gets to be.

It can be so energizing and fun to use these tools! There are too few opportunities in life to feel positive in some of the sad and serious jobs we perform. Tragedy surrounds us in health care, and it is easy to be sucked into the sorrowful side of life. Using these fun and energizing instant teaching tools can provide an opportunity for a balance of feelings for ourselves and our learners. What a great outlet and contribution to those in our field! Feel positive about the job you do as educator. We deliver much more than information to our audiences; we provide them with a positive and fun outlet, while gaining new knowledge and skills. Be proud. Enjoy!

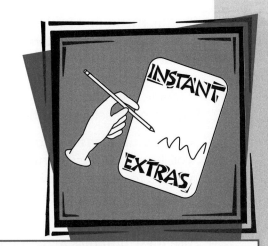

PART 6

INSTANT EXTRAS

Surprise! Here is an extra section meant to offer you some fun and whimsical building blocks for the creation of visuals. Created by my terrific friend and multitalented artist Lori Backer, these instant visuals are designed to add a little "extra" to your teaching session. By design, these graphics provide you with a teaching tool to help you deliver your message with a light-hearted approach. They provide a little fun and sometimes even laughter for professionals who face the stark realities of their profession daily.

Incorporating visuals to introduce or conclude a mini-lecture allows you to present key learning points in a most effective way. Use these visuals to grab your audience's attention. Remember, over 80% of the average population access information visually, so tap into this mode of learning!

Use these graphics to design overheads, slides, computer screens, handout pages, and flip chart pages. To create slides for use with computerized presentation software, simply scan the page of your choice and use it as a template for your slide. You can add your content or lecture material in the center of the graphic and have an appealing and interesting ready-to-use visual presentation. When creating a handout, choose a graphic and use it as a border for page layout and add your content outline or key lecture material. The appropriate border picture and word combine to act as a low attention-level reinforcement tool and overall unifying element. Invite your learners to color the message-related graphic, if desired.

If you are artistically gifted, you can copy the border design on flip chart pages and add your content information. Display the completed content pages in your teaching environment, and you have a creative content reinforcement tool. These graphic templates can also be used to decorate educational bulletin boards.

Feel free to use the graphics and add your own words in the borders whenever necessary. Let your imagination play with the elements of each of these pages. Be creative and inspire your audience. Last but not least, I want to point out one of my favorite templates. It's the last template in this section, and it always brings a smile to anyone in our industry who views it. Use it often and ENJOY!

BILL OF RIGHTS

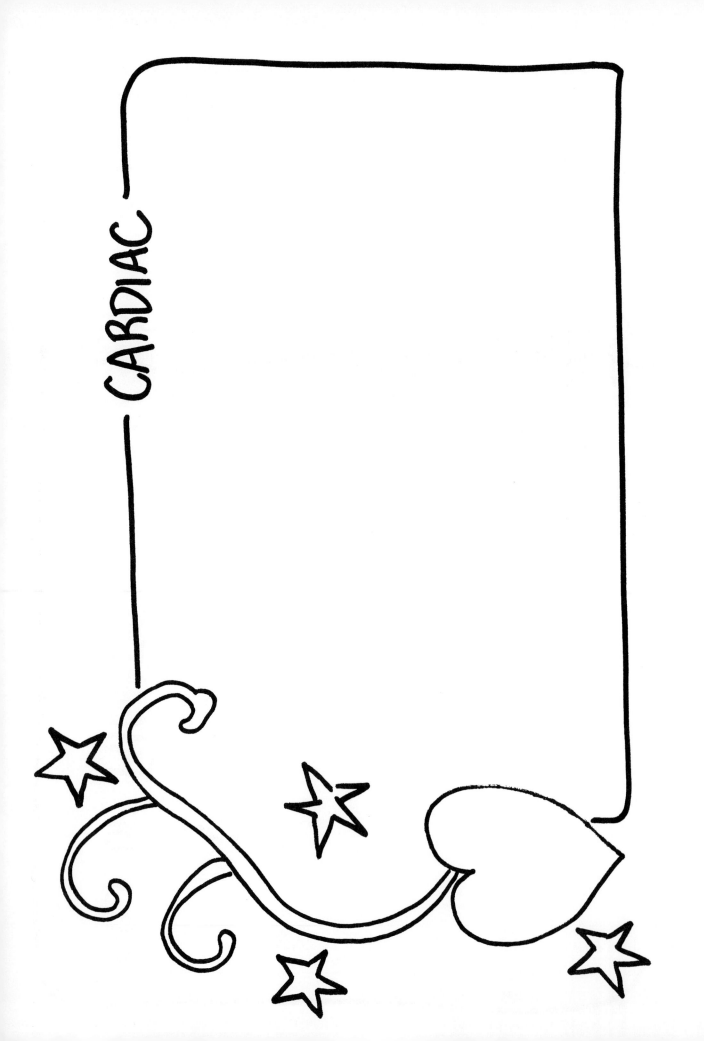

CARDIAC

FIRE SAFETY

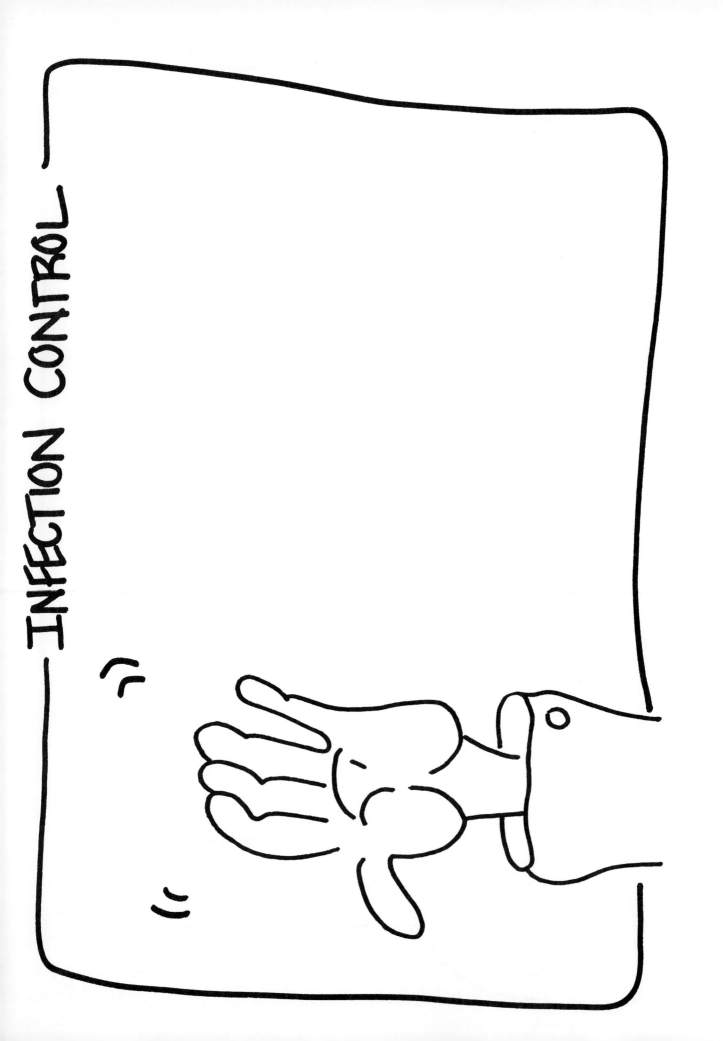

INFECTION CONTROL

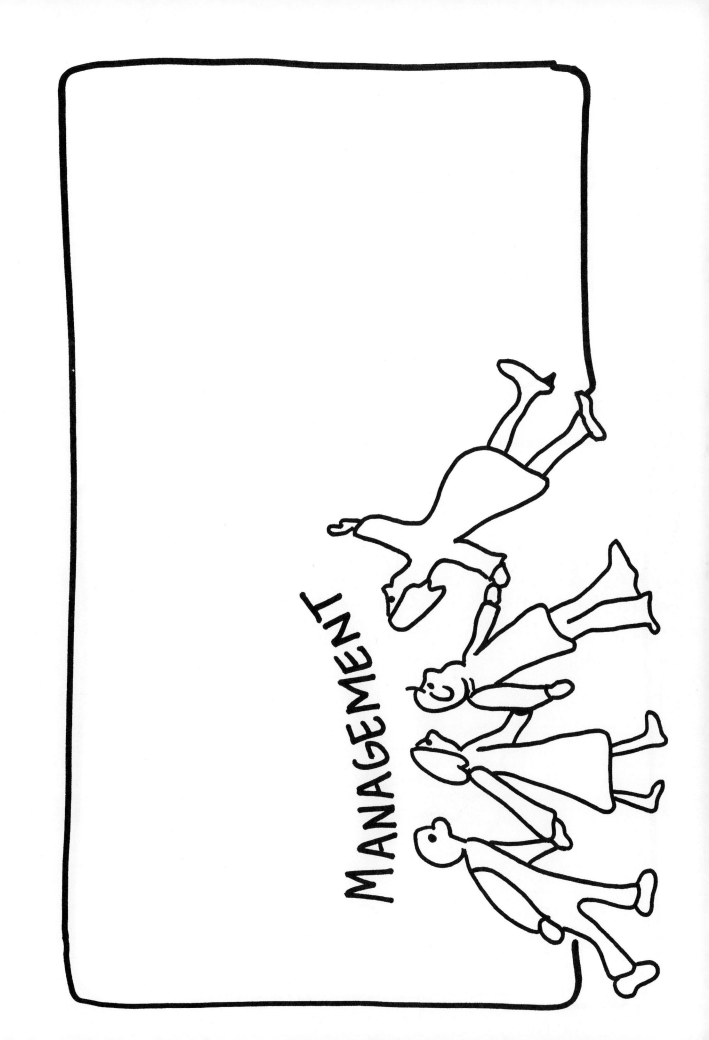

MANAGEMENT

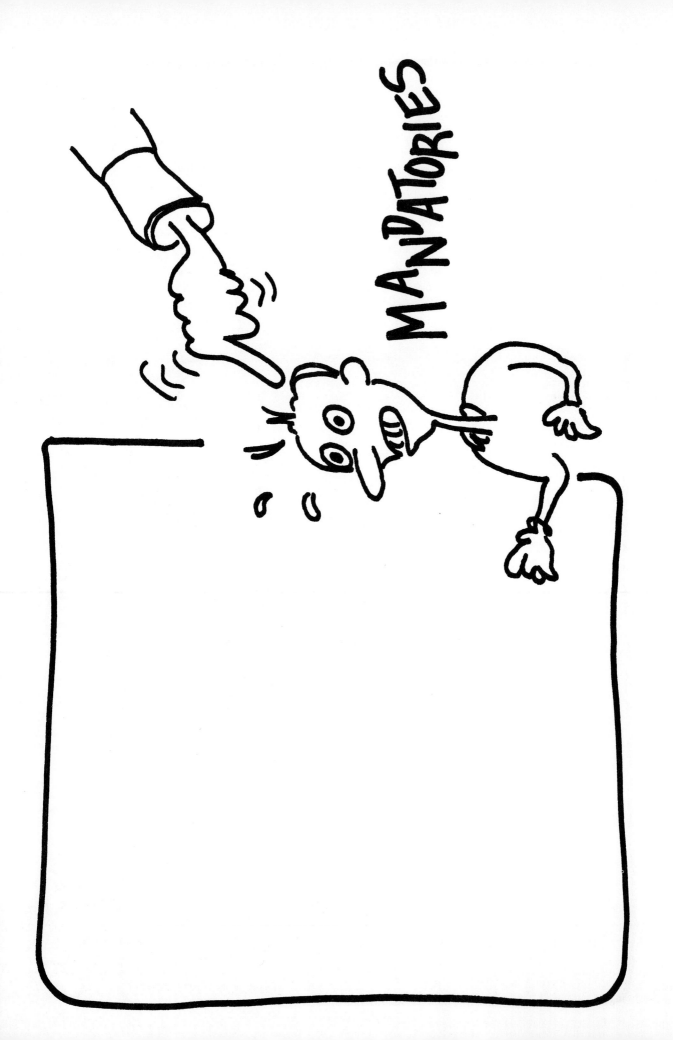

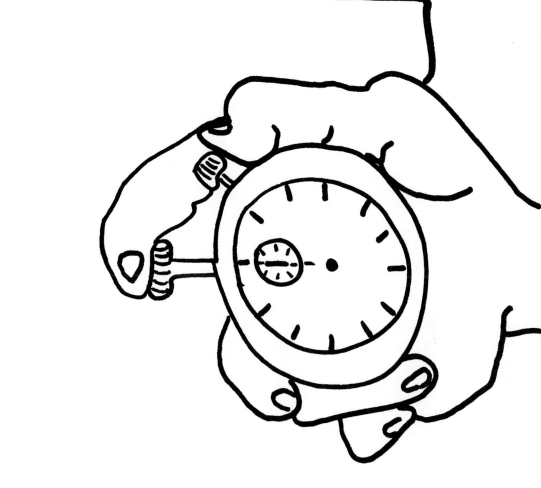

MEDICATIONS

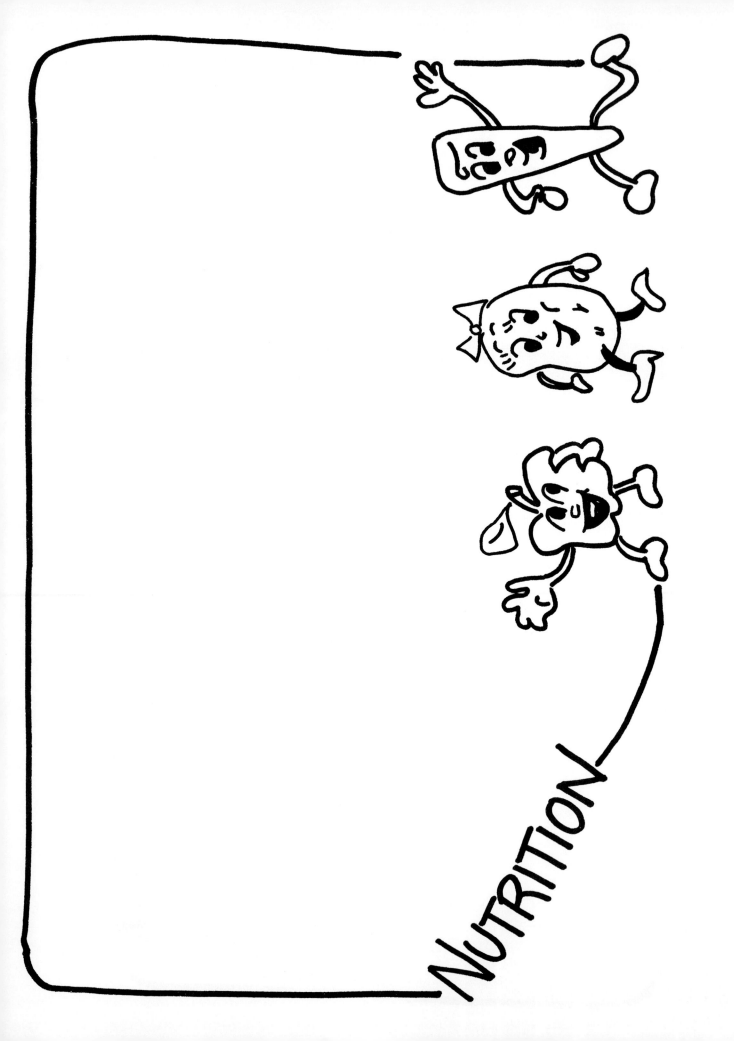

NUTRITION

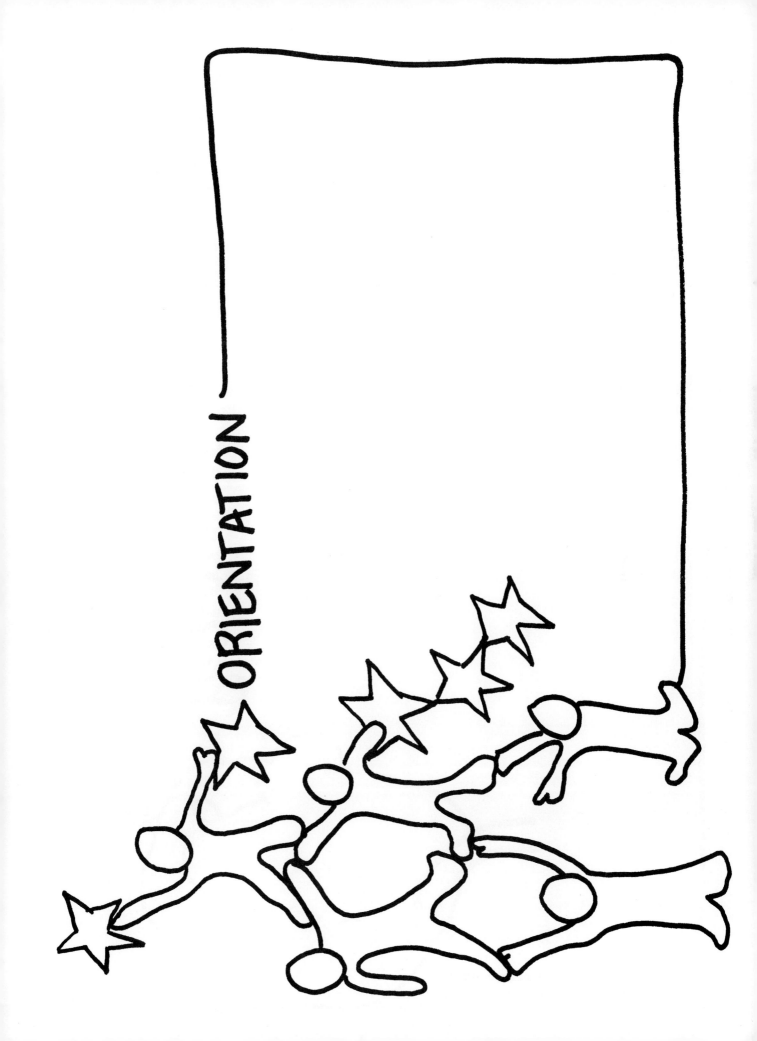

ORIENTATION

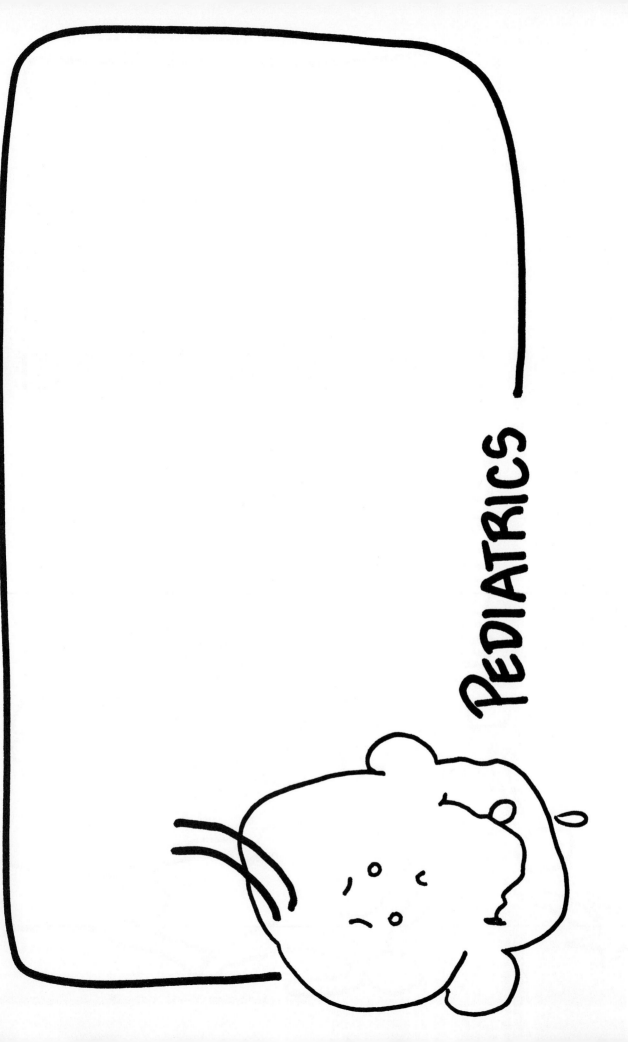

PEDIATRICS

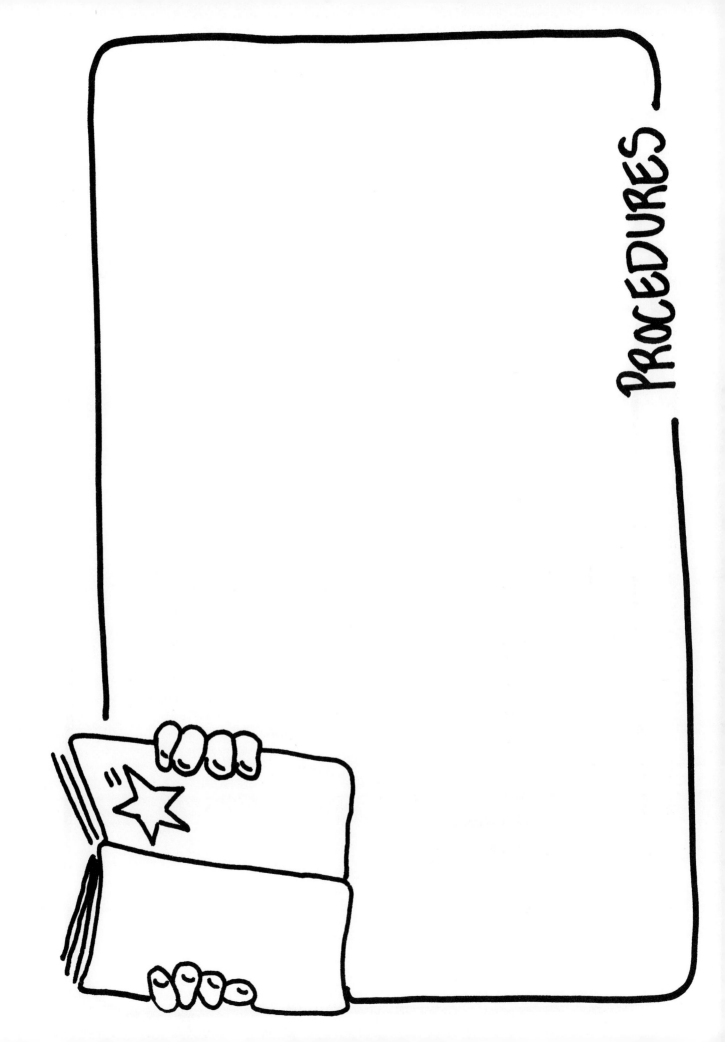

PROCEDURES

SAFETY

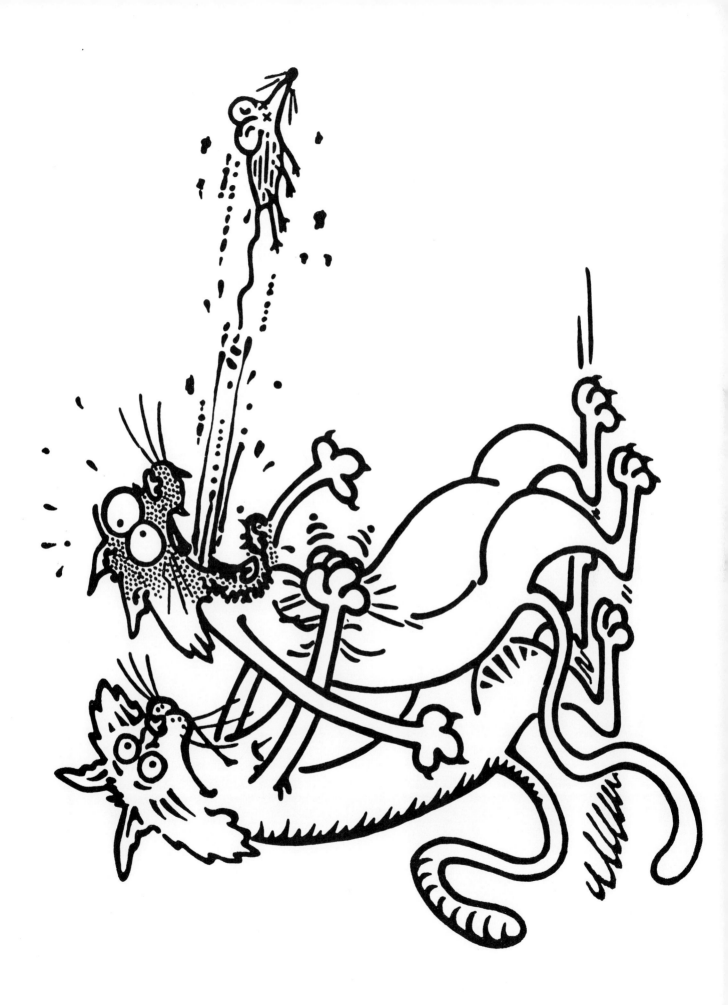

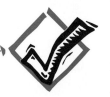

If you have an idea that you are willing to share and would like to have included in Volume 3 of *Instant Teaching Tools for Healthcare Educators,* please complete the form on the following page. Feel free to copy the form and submit as many ideas as you would like!

Please send your ideas to:
Michele Deck
c/o Mosby
Attn: Nursing Editorial
11830 Westline Industrial Drive
St. Louis, MO 63146

or contact Michele directly via the Internet at:
gamesinc4@aol.com

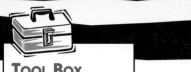

Length of time

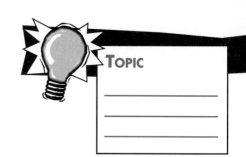

TOPIC

_____
_____
_____

_____
(Suggested Activity Title)

TOOL BOX
(Tools required
to implement
activity)

_____
_____
_____
_____
_____
_____
_____

Preparation:

_____
_____
_____
_____
_____
_____
_____
_____

Implementation:

_____
_____
_____
_____
_____
_____
_____
_____
_____
_____
_____
_____
_____
_____
_____
_____
_____
_____
_____
_____

**EDUCATOR
SECRETS:**

_____
_____
_____
_____

By: _____
(Source or author of activity)

Bibliography

Deck M, Silva J: *Getting adults motivated, enthusiastic and satisfied,* Minneapolis, 1990, Creative Training Techniques International.

Deck M, Silva J: *Getting adults motivated, enthusiastic and satisfied, volume two,* Minneapolis, 1997, Creative Training Techniques International.

Pike RW: *Creative training techniques handbook,* Minneapolis, 1996, Lakewood Books.